PAIN

We Need a New Definition

Rudy Kachmann M.D.

Rudy Kachmann M.D.
Published by Rudy Kachmann, M.D.

www.KachmannMindBody.com
Copyright © 2012Rudy Kachmann M.D.

ISBN-10: 1478216603
EAN-13: 9781478216605
Printed in the United States of America

CONTENTS

PREFACE

Pain centers: a growing national scandal

I just cannot take it anymore. For years I have witnessed the abusive, inappropriate, probably fraudulent, addictive, overly aggressive treatment of chronic pain problems by pain centres. They are habituating and addicting people right and left. There are many tragic stories. I see these people in the office week after week. We doctors all know it. People are dying.

The medical society, at local, state, and national levels, does little about it. The pain societies are driven by money and are not fixing the obvious problems.

People pick up the paper and see national stories weekly. Around December 2011 in Scioto County, Ohio, all pain clinics were closed by the state. The Drug Enforcement Administration said that Southern Ohio County is one of the worst places in the country for painkiller abuse. A county grand jury indicted two providers with charges including engaging in corrupt activity, drug trafficking, and drug possession. The people involved were charged with engaging in corrupt activity, conspiracy to engage in corrupt activity, funding drug trafficking, and permitting drug abuse. Stopping the abuse of powerful prescription painkillers is a top priority for Ohio officials. In 2007, drug overdoses led by an increase in prescription painkiller addictions, surpassing car crashes as the leading cause of accidental death in Ohio. It is a trend also seen in several other states, with fifteen thousand deaths in the country.

In May Gov. John Kasich signed into law a bill cracking down on pain management clinics dubbed "narcotic mills" by their critics and blamed by health officials for contributing to thousands of overdose deaths in Ohio each year. The State Board of Pharmacy requires pain clinics to be licensed as distributors of dangerous drugs.

That said, the state has actually suspended the prescription-writing powers of some physicians in a part of southern Ohio plagued by painkiller abuse. More than 1,300 people died from accidental narcotic overdose in 2009 in Ohio, according to the most recent data from the Ohio Department of Health. The number of deaths from overdoses has more than quadrupled since 1999, when the state recorded 327 accidental narcotic overdose deaths, according to the department.

Seventy deaths from medical narcotics occurred in our surrounding counties in Fort Wayne last year, essentially the same number as the year before. My friend's beautiful daughter died from a physician prescription from a pain centre. There are probably over fifteen thousand deaths nationally from physician narcotic prescriptions. Let us face it: it is a war. What is even worse, the taxpayers are paying the bill for the procedures and addictive narcotics. Medicare and Medicaid are paying about ninety percent of the bill. I reviewed the latter estimate with the director of a holistic pain clinic, and he said that figure was accurate. In other words, the government is paying for the procedures and medicines that addict people, and then they send them home in a taxi paid for by the government, after which they have to treat the chronic ailments from their procedures and medications. Most of those people, of course, will be unemployed and pay no taxes. The Medicaid taxi driver told me the whole story and I will have a chapter of his words further in the book. What a deal! I am blowing the whistle on this fraud.

This book will explain chronic pain so people can understand it, and then I will expose the mistreatment of it. Finally, I will give my recommendations to correct the situation. It is a war out there!

Birth of the Baby: A History of Pain Clinics

We learned a lot about narcotics, especially morphine, which is derived from opium, in the 1800s. It was especially popular during the First World War. We created three hundred thousand soldier addicts; addiction was called "soldier's disease." Opium had been used for thousands of years, but its metabolite morphine was discovered in the 1800s. Around the turn of the century (1900), patients and physicians thought morphine and cocaine were medical and recreational drugs. Famous psychiatrist

Dr. Sigmund Freud and renowned surgeon Dr. William Stewart Halsted were regular users of these medications, as recently described in a popular book. Around World War I, the medical profession recognized morphine's intense habituation and addicting potential. The word "addiction" was coined at that time and generally meant overwhelming high, severe craving and willingness to break the law to get more medicine. Physicians no longer considered opiates benign and realized there was a high risk of so-called "iatrogenic addiction."

In 1914 the federal government passed the Harrison Narcotics Tax Act, the nation's first drug law. It was a tax and a record-keeping statute rather than law enforcement. But the US Supreme Court issued an opinion in 1919 that interpreted the Harrison Act as also barring the prescriptions of narcotics to patients addicted to them. Today that law seems to be totally ignored by many pain centers. They may claim they did not know the patient was an addict, but it's not hard to tell that in my experience. All you have to do is look at the government site "INSPECT," or get a blood test, or look at the people in the waiting room.

By the late 1930s more than twenty-five thousand doctors had been charged with offenses relative to the Harrison Act. Morphine was then largely given for cancer patients, appropriately so.

In 1973 the pain movement became pregnant. Three hundred fifty researchers from around the world gathered near Seattle for the creation of the International Association for the Study of Pain.

Morphine gets its name from Morpheus, the Greek god of sleep. Morphine, an opiate, became very popular. The Sloan-Kettering Cancer Institute in New York, a great place, started using morphine IV drips for pain control in cancer patients. It worked very well and still does. We now use it a great deal in hospice situations, especially for advanced cases generally leading to death. In the early days, doctors gave morphine continuously in the blood instead of intermittently. That gave much better pain relief to patients with advanced cancer. The hospice movement started in London in the 1980s. Very few cancer patients became addicted because of the real pain and their shortened lifespan. I'm sure a few became addicted who survived their cancer or lived a long time. Generally holistic methods were not used that much at that time at Sloan-Kettering, although they are now.

The trouble started when providers started using morphine for noncancer, chronic, long-term pain problems. The addiction rate was not one percent as believed, but much higher. It was discovered that many of the noncancer patients with chronic pain actually were depressed, anxious, and hopeless; many also had work-related job dissatisfaction, and some were seeking disability. War veterans are paid more when they have more pain. Lawsuits from accidents often depended on the amount of pain a person is experiencing. Those in greater pain are more likely to get workman's comp, Social Security, or disability, and you can imagine how much trouble that starts.

Throughout the 1970s multiple disciplines were used for nonaddictive pain problems, including exercise, diet, yoga, music, massages, etc. The insurance companies did not pay well for these, although they worked well and caused no addiction.

A pain cancer specialist named Dr. Kanner thought physicians had "opiophobia," a term used by the pain management movement to describe doctors who were afraid to prescribe opioids for pain, thinking they would starve the baby, but this only made it grow faster. Dr. Kanner was a researcher who studied with Dr. Russell Portenoy in New York. Dr. Portenoy was working at the Albert Einstein College of Medicine in 1981. He is the father of the baby, although no genetic testing has been done. Kathleen Foley is another important figure in the pain field and also worked with Dr. Portenoy.

Dr. Portenoy's idea was simple and optimistic: a subpopulation of chronic pain patients might benefit greatly from long-term use of powerful narcotic drugs which already had been shown to be fairly safe in cancer patients. That indeed was his experience. He concluded that opioid maintenance narcotic therapy could be a safe alternative to surgery or no treatment for patients with "chronic non-malignant pain."

He didn't define what non-malignant pain was, though, and that was a big mistake. There are different types of chronic pain, and the type makes a lot of difference when considering narcotic prescriptions. There's a lot of difference between true neuropathic pain and centralized brain pain— what I called "Metabolic Pain" (centralized brain pain) (centralized brain pain)," a term I coined to describe pain that's based on hopelessness, anxiety, fear, depression, and the bumps and bruises of your life. As far as I'm concerned, these patients should not be given narcotics, as they are prone to become addicts. They need the dopamine and serotonin to feel good. They can get it through food, sex, or narcotics, as well as through numerous holistic methods like music, exercise, etc.

Dr. Kathleen Foley and Dr. Portenoy wrote their opinion and were the mother and father of the "pain baby" that was born around that time. All this history is described in detail by the "baby war" called N.M.C.P. (nonmalignant chronic pain) in *New York Times* reporter Barry Meier's great book, *Painkiller*. I highly recommend you read it for more detail. When I received it in the mail from Amazon, I read the whole thing straight through the night after a hard day's work. I just couldn't put it down and I am rereading it again right now, especially now that I've written a book myself called *The Fraud of Chronic Pain*.

I've been facing these pain people for a number of years and fully realize they are, the creation of the medical community and it must stop. I've seen many patients who've suffered severe neurological damage from cardiac arrest and respiratory arrest, which often lead to death. I see it every week, and every week I try to change the system through contacting government agencies, lecturing, and writing.

Dr. Portenoy published over a hundred papers and lectured throughout the country promoting his ideas, paid for largely by drug companies. Some people would call him an evangelist. They may call me an evangelist too, and that's fine with me. I'm going to save a lot of lives. Hardly anybody dies from pain, but they are dying in the tens of thousands from narcotic prescriptions.

Portenoy was promoting a drug-based approach, the opposite of mine, a mind-body approach that includes things like diet, exercise, yoga, music, and massage. Pain can be improved with the Portenoy approach, but the patient's function is seriously impaired. If people have any doubt about it, just sit in the waiting room of a few pain clinics, like my patients and I have done many times. You feel like you're sitting in the waiting room of a concentration camp or drug house. Just open your eyes and look at the people staring straight ahead, smelling horribly, most looking destitute, and many with tattoos, as the pain of tattooing secretes endorphins and makes them feel better for a little while.

The loss of functionality, I think, is the biggest reason that I do not like the Portenoy approach. The majority of these patients cannot and many will not work in the future. Once they're addicted, their chances of getting rid of that monkey on their back is maybe about ten percent. Some of my psychiatrist friends think it's only five percent or less. You can see why I am so passionate about prevention. Short-term use of a narcotic can get a person to work sometimes, but if they take them for a time, they become tolerant of the medication and doses will have to be increased, pushing them down the road of addiction and habituation. Many become addicted, not a mere one percent, as Dr. Portenoy and Dr. Foley originally claimed.

Loss of functionality is the wolf in the henhouse. As we mentioned, just sit in the waiting room of a pain clinic. It's horrifying listening to the stories. Many speak about selling the medication as soon as they get it because they are economically stressed. Ninety percent of patients aren't functioning, and many are on Medicaid because they are broke. Medicaid does not have deductibles; the government will pay for a taxi to pick these addicted people up from their houses, for the visit to the pain doctor and for the medication, and for the taxi to take them home. Most are on Medicaid and Social Security disability while the rest of us are working. Read the story of my eighteen-year-old patient further on in the book. He couldn't stand to be in the waiting room of the pain clinic because of the way it Looked, smelled and the activity going on there, Even a child as young as he recognized the problem.

Large crowds started attending Dr. Portenoy's lectures and a new industry was born—the pain clinic. The baby had arrived and no one recognized it was disabled. Everyone thought reducing chronic pain no matter the cause was a laudable goal, and that was a big mistake! Sure, some people with neuropathic pain were treated more effectively, as well as patients with cancer pain, but that was not the majority of the cases. Very few of the patients were functioning normally, even though they could've worked if other methods had been used. A "pain industrial complex" arose in my town and all over the country. If you want to see a horror movie, go to about a half a dozen waiting rooms of the pain clinics and you'll see what

I mean. The doctors who practice in other specialties across the hall from pain clinics complain about it every day in the doctor's lounge. Some of these pain patients have even invaded their offices, and they've had to lock up when they go to lunch.

Pain management was a new specialty in the early years and huge crowds attended Dr. Portenoy's lectures. Other trips and nice vacations were paid for by the pharmaceutical industry. He provided pain activists with the data and statistics they needed on the media, social, and medical front. They needed food (opioids) to feed the baby.

A number of scientific papers were published in the mid-1980s. Dr. Portenoy claimed the low addiction rates—three hundred thousand soldiers in the First World War— were misleading and represented a biased opinion. He said the addiction rate is only one percent, but this was based on little data. Dr. Portenoy pointed to three scientific papers as his proof. They were quietly adapted by the pain management system and to help promote them. In 1980 the *New England Journal of Medicine*, a well-known journal that used to have a great reputation, published an article about narcotic use and hospital patients. The second study appeared in 1977 in the *Journal of Headaches*. The third study was published in in the *Pain Journal* in May of 1982, reviewing the pain of burn patients. Portenoy claimed the studies proved only about one percent of these patients ever became addicted. What he didn't say was that there is the tremendous difference between hospitalized patients who generally are there for a good reason and the general public showing up at a pain clinic without an acute illness, many suffering from Metabolic Pain (centralized brain pain) (centralized brain pain) (centralized brain pain) (centralized brain pain). Many of the latter have no idea why they hurt. Clinic staff just asked what the level of the pain was and gave them the medicine they wanted—Vicodin, morphine, OxyContin, Fentanyl, etc. That's a good way to build an addict.

Purdue Pharma LP would use these statistics and also claim that the addiction rates were low, promoting MS Contin and oxycodone.

Dr. Portenoy covered his trail by saying medical staff must take an addiction history and really know the case before prescribing. Unfortunately, this recommendation has been greatly ignored by many pain centers. I see it every week.

In the *Journal of Pain and Symptom Management,* an obscure journal that most doctors never read, Dr. Portenoy spoke about the aforementioned issues. Out on the road, though, he told a different story. Most providers get the information from road shows, newspapers, TV, and meetings paid for by the pharmaceutical companies. The journals above were not quoted. I still remember meeting the OxyContin saleslady about ten years ago. The reason I remember her she was the most gorgeous thing I'd seen in years and I have to be proud of myself that I didn't fall for her sales pitch. I remember she visited my office two or three times without my invitation.

Portenoy told the *New York Times* that there was a growing literature showing that the drugs can be used for a long time for benign pain conditions with few side effects, and that addiction and habituation are not a problem. He said that at the same time his article appeared in the *Journal of Pain and Symptom Management,* which was a lot more sober. Sadly, the majority of doctors never heard of it. They certainly did not hand out copies of it at the meetings when he spoke, meetings that were largely paid for by drug companies.

There is no question that pain centers are needed, especially for the treatment of pain for cancer patients, neuropathic pain, and some elderly patients, for whom pain treatment had not been what it should be—at least, that's what they all say. But is that really the case? I don't remember seeing a lot of suffering among the patients. Perhaps they were a little slow in the hospital, and now that pain is the fifth vital sign, those things are addressed more quickly. The nurse never seems to ask about the cause of one's pain, it's based on the word of the patient—"What is the level of your pain on a scale of 0 to 10?" You can see where problem is. I listen to the patient's complaints. It's actually the addicted patient who is difficult to deal with. They don't stop giving me a hard time unless I give into their request. Believe me, I've been through it.

I've heard the term "barbaric" used to describe the way pain used to be treated. I don't agree with that. The government did get involved with the creation of the fifth vital sign. Some patients have even started suing doctors for not addressing their pain. Can you imagine what an addicted person might do? They have been very difficult to deal with, but I don't even blame them. They can't help it; it's a medical provider who addicted them in the first place. That is who I am critical of, the nurses and doctors in the emergency room who ask about pain level and then treat it with narcotics. You can see the mistakes resulting from that. You can see the problems that can occur in the emergency room. Just recently two of my patients were given Dilaudid for no good reason, simply because the doctor asked about the level of their pain. He said, "Well, I can give you a Fentanyl patch to take care of you for the weekend." Guess what? A few days later I checked on my patient and found out she had sold the Fentanyl on the street and was seeking another prescription in my office. I did have a talk with that doctor. Of course some of the patients in the ER do have acute pain, other than cancer patients, who require stronger medications.

States like Texas have even passed laws to ensure that stronger pain medications are used for patients, urging medical providers to write the prescriptions. I feel the threat of patients every day when I tell them that narcotics are not appropriate. I encourage physicians, especially in the office and E.R. to check Indiana's program called INSPECT. That will tell providers if the patient has been doctor shopping, which is typical of the painkiller addict. The idea of the INSPECT system was to catch pain mills, overprescribing doctors, and patients who are abusing the system. The American Medical Association tried to prevent these systems from coming into place, totally ignoring the habitual addiction and increasing deaths. There have been a lot of stories about this in newspapers from Florida and Kentucky. Lee County, Kentucky, has had an especially big problem. I actually think Indiana has been quite reasonable in establishing the INSPECT system which I think should be national, and I personally think they should periodically audit pain clinics throughout the country. They make a lot of money and that is something that they have to put up with.

In the mid-1990s many articles appeared in national publications claiming, falsely, about the under treatment of pain. Hardly anybody dies from pain. Many countries don't allow narcotics to be used at all, only in some patients with cancer.

Time magazine published an article called the "Morphine Myth," and it was the dumbest article I've ever read. They did not do their research. The journals, newspapers, and TV miss the main story—the drug companies. But Barry Meier from the *New York Times* certainly didn't miss it. He chillingly chronicles pharmaceutical companies, especially Purdue Pharma LP, in great detail. I commend him for that. The company knew the problems of addiction. The three brothers who formed the company in New York City have completely ruined their reputations as far as I am concerned. Of course I doubt they care since they're all dead. But I suspect their children are running it now because it's a private company.

Industry monies supported research by investigators like Kathy Foley and Russell Portenoy, and virtually every pain manager was paid a consultant fee for speaking engagements for a narcotic product. Money poured into the Pain Society and the American Academy of Pain Medicine. The two societies represent the pain doctors.

Dr. David Joe Ranson's group at the University of Wisconsin received a lot of money also. They were called the Pain and Policy Study Group. Other pharmaceutical companies included Knoll Pharmaceuticals, McNeill, and Purdue Pharma.

Purdue Pharma gave hundreds of thousands of dollars to the Wisconsin Group.

Pain clinics exploded in places like Lee County, Kentucky, in West Virginia, Florida, Georgia, Ohio, and frankly all over the country.

Kathleen Foley called the drug companies "allies in education." What a joke. "Colleagues in death" would be a better term.

The APS, American Pain Society, should be called the American Pharmaceutical Society. Barry Meier, the *New York Times* reporter, said, and I agree, that the addiction rate is incorrect. I suspect it's more like thirty percent or maybe even higher. Certainly if people were to visit some the pain clinics, I would guess they'd put the estimate around seventy to eighty percent.

Clearly it was Dr. Portenoy who was the main promoter. He even visited Purdue Pharma to encourage them to make a long-lasting narcotic like MS Contin, which resulted in OxyContin. He was looking for long-term narcotic medication. I'm sure he was sincere in his efforts, but he was just plain wrong in what it produced in the end. We already had medicine to treat the cancer patients; we didn't need the stronger MS Contin and oxycodone for non-malignant pain problems. They should just admit it and move on to better treatment of pain and try to undo some of the horrible damage. Unfortunately, many of the pain patients are addicted now across the nation, and the odds of breaking that addiction to opioids is probably around ten percent. I would say a good ninety percent of these people are not functioning and don't have a job. When you look at people in the waiting room of pain clinics, you can clearly see that hardly any of them could possibly be working. I understand that ninety percent of these patients are on Medicaid, which tells you the story of what's going on in their lives.

The leaders, the father and mother of the pain industry in the US, must admit their mistakes and work even harder, like Dr. Ballantyne from the state of Washington has, to undo what's going on. She admitted she was mistaken when she thought like Dr. Portenoy. I congratulate her. I don't know everything, but I hope I've always had the integrity to do something different when I was wrong!

Unfortunately, the baby "pain centers" was born and is disabled. We know who the parents are. They must help us to take care of it and help develop a proper treatment for non-malignant chronic pain problems. The "baby" needs to be born again and have better parents.

The Awakening

The *New York Times* published a great article by Barry Meier on April 9, 2012.

To me he hit the nail on the head, and maybe he partially awakened the pain centers and providers to the point that the treatment of chronic pain is generally dead wrong. The state of Washington, after burying forty people from narcotic prescription overdoses, woke up to the problem and tried to do something about it. At first they pointed out the problem to the medical providers, but that accomplished little, probably because there was a lot of money in it. So they quickly passed a state law stating that if the blood level of a patient exceeds 120 mg of morphine or its equivalent, they are to be referred to a pain center physician. In my experience with pain centers, that's like putting the fox in the chicken coop. they'll make a permanent customer out of them. The majority of pain centers have no nonaddictive holistic treatment in their arsenal. Injections, implants, stimulators, and narcotics are their ballgame and the money this generates.

We have to figure out a better way. Pain centers are the promoters of pain treatments involving the body, and many of the patients are habitually addicted to the opiate prescriptions. Ohio is considering doing the same thing as the state of Washington. Hopefully I can talk to them and help them design a better way. As we know, there have been too many complications and deaths from narcotic prescriptions in the state of Ohio. The number of deaths exceeds that of car accidents now.

Awareness by providers is improving in the state of Washington and they are having some success, but with the fox in the chicken coop, things will only improve to a certain point and may even get worse. Everybody knows where the money is. Dr. Russell K. Ballantyne, a pain specialist for the state of Washington, changed her mind about how pain should be treated. She noticed when she examined hospital patients that their skin appeared to be sensitized from the narcotic medications. That is a well-known phenomenon to most psychiatrists and addiction-treating specialists, including myself. I saw a patient like that recently—I could not touch this patient without him jumping, and his mind was so excitable that he acted like he was going to punch me. His pain specialist had increased his morphine to 45 mg the day before. Where do you think he's heading? I hope he wakes up tomorrow! I spent a lot of time with him, but I will tell you, speaking to a habitually addicted patient is like talking to a wall. They will only leave the office when they have their prescription in hand. They are extremely unreasonable. You have to remember, they are not thinking logically, they need that overwhelming high to just feel normal.

Dr. Ballantyne said that about fifteen years ago we liberalized our prescription procedures for opiates and opiates; unfortunately we were all dead wrong in doing it. She says she changed her mind and awakened to the tremendous problems we have created in treating chronic pain. At least, she admitted it in the *New York Times* article. Dr. Russell Portenoy from New York City is still thinking the old way and hasn't changed his mind. He thinks we should just pay more attention to this problem and that nothing is especially wrong. This type of thinking has resulted in fifteen thousand deaths this year from opiate prescriptions in the US. I personally think Dr. Portenoy needs to spend a few days and nights in about ten different pain centers. Just sitting in the waiting rooms will give him plenty of education.

The long-term use of opiates for chronic pain is fairly new. Until fifteen years ago the drugs were largely used for postoperative care, major injuries, or end-of-life care. Isn't it strange that in many countries of the world opiates are not used at all and the people seem to have good lives? We have created a pain culture, and the government is paying for this. Ninety percent of these patients use Medicaid, and this is paving the streets of pain and death and gold. They were horribly wrong, in my opinion, and it has created many disabilities and continues to kill people in the thousands. Pain does not kill people, opiates do, and your government is paying for it!

Time Release: The Pot of Gold

The Purdue Pharma LP pharmaceutical company bought a small company in Britain that had developed the technology of time release for a drug called MS Contin. In other words, if you took a pill, it would last twelve hours instead of four. This was very helpful for the cancer patient. They might sleep through the night. In the late 1900s, the people in the street discovered that crushing MS Contin and oxycodone produced extreme highs, as well as overwhelming cravings because of its purity. The drug was not mixed in with anything else like aspirin or Tylenol. It was all hydrocodone or morphine as a basic chemical. The pharmaceutical companies didn't count on the people on the street to figure out how to sell and use the medication; however, all you had to do is to chew it or crush it, so it is hard to believe that they did not anticipate what was happening early in the game. Before that the companies had promoted the time-release medication as more safe and with less chance of addiction. That was either a big mistake or frankly a big old lie. A Canadian study actually revealed that MS Contin, a time-release morphine, was appearing in the inner city drug market. They learned about that from drug dealers. MS was crushed, liquefied, and injected for a great high. They called it "peelers." The 10 mg tablets were green; the 30 mg tablets were purple. OxyContin could be chewed up and swallowed. They found it only takes five days for many people to get addicted to these medications. That is why it is dangerous for pain doctors to give patients a choice of drugs like morphine, methadone, or OxyContin, as you will read about in the upcoming section "The Struggle," which describes a horrific situation, including death, disability, and lifetime addiction. This goes on in the majority of pain centers in the nation on a daily basis. Addiction can occur quickly, and originally all the patient had was a backache and even that was questionable. Four pain centers did the exact same thing—injected the patient without a clear diagnosis and then gave her multiple highly addicting medications.

Physician-induced dependency and addiction became common in the early 2000s and is still common today. I see it all the time. Yes, even using a narcotic as recommended, without crushing it, can result in addiction, and the rate is a lot higher than one percent. Pain clinics are the biggest promoters of injections or procedures on the spine, and when these don't work, the narcotic prescriptions begin. Epidural blocks and injections act as the key that unlocks the door to the narcotics and many times a lifetime of suffering when administered to noncancer patients.

Thousands die every year from overdoses of OxyContin, methadone, in combination with Xanax, diazepam, and other drugs.

WHAT IS PAIN

A sensation—Snoopy says it's when it hurts. A feeling, a perception, an emotion...it varies greatly. Pain comes from the *paena*, "to suffer." Males and females appreciate pain differently; females are a lot more sensitive to pain, thought to be related to their lack of endorphins, possibly related to estrogen. There are different perceptions of pain among races, cultures, ethnic groups, children, and adults.

One hundred million people have some sort of a pain problem daily. We spend probably $100 billion a year on pain medication, not counting injections and operations and manipulations, a huge cost.

Pain represents fifty to eighty percent of doctor visits daily. Pain is affected by biology, physiology, and psychology. Many pain specialists say we are undertreating pain. I say we are over treating pain, big time. The national and local news recently reported that more people are dying from addiction to physician-issued narcotic prescriptions than from the drugs from Colombia and Mexico. Think we have a serious problem? Who is the criminal here?

There is no good test for pain. That is the problem. They talk about functional MRIs, but the reality of usefulness is a long way off, maybe decades. When a person's blood sugar is 500, we know they're diabetic. When people say their pain is an 8, we can't be one hundred percent sure about anything. Are they a drug seeker? Pain specialists will say, "The word of the patient is the gold standard in the treatment of chronic pain." I say they are dreaming. A diagnosis of "cause" should be the gold standard to avoid the tremendous amount of overtreatment with addictive drugs, which is what we are witnessing. Very few people will die from the lack of treatment of chronic pain, but a huge number are dying yearly from narcotics prescribed for unclear reasons. A lot of providers confuse drug withdrawal, tolerance, drug dependency, and drug addiction with the need for pain medication. The majority of chronic pain patients are looking for the quick fix, and we are willing to give it to them because of a confused state of "the gold standard of pain care." The real problem is that many providers don't understand the difference between acute and non-neuropathic chronic pain. Acute pain is a protective mechanism of the body. Pain or pleasure is what keeps life going. That's nature. Acute pain tells people something is wrong, maybe life-threatening. It may tell people what part of the body is involved and leads to a diagnosis and a cure. The pain goes away and no further medication as needed. The cycle of pain medication has a beginning and an end. The likelihood of habituation or addiction is extremely small. The broken bone is fixed and the pain is probably gone for good. A beginning and an end have occurred. Acute pain can be lifesaving. Chronic pain, pain lasting longer than six months, is another story altogether. Don't confuse the two, though the medical profession does every day. Chronic pain is divided into neuropathic, non-neuropathic, nociceptive, and idiopathic pain, or pain of unclear diagnosis. Neuropathic means pain from nerve damage, as from an amputated leg, diabetic neuropathy, pinched nerves, etc. It means that damage has occurred to a nerve. This type of pain represents maybe twenty percent of chronic pain. Some of these problems may need strong medications or injections for a period of time. But the medications lose effectiveness after a number of months, and narcotics don't work well for neuropathic pain. Then again, some of these patients need to be on antidepressants, narcotics, and anti-inflammatory medications for a number of months and some for years. Mind-healing techniques, yoga, meditation, massage, and exercise have great value yet are generally not tried enough. They should be the first line of defense, rather than addictive drugs, because drugs change the brain circuitry. Once people change their brain circuitry, the chances of getting rid of the pain become slimmer because of tolerance, habituation, and addiction.

The larger category of pain by far is the chronic pain of unclear diagnosis. No clear nerve damage, no clear impairment, but the patient says, "I hurt." Many of these patients have had a dozen MRIs, CT scans, nerve blocks, and surgeries to no avail. What causes it? A combination of biological, physiological, and psychological factors. The patients need to be asked Dr. Rudy's pain questions. These will be listed in a chapter by that name before treatment begins to avoid addiction. Psychology plays a huge role in these cases. The medical community is having a financial windfall with this huge group of psychologically dependent pain people. We could build a large city with their numbers, unfortunately. The majority are suffering, probably not working, and collecting a lot of money in disability payments.

The human body is also involved with this financial windfall of fraud. It's giving people pain but nothing life-threatening is going on. They're plagued by it, spend a lot of money on it, can't sleep, become anxious and depressed, and they don't even know why they're hurting. They may spend their lifetime on it. A significant amount of it may have been started by the medications they were given. Chronic pain can be a false signal, or it could be warning that there is something wrong in one's life, but no single test can be done to prove it. Social problems, family problems, negative thinking, unemployment, an accident, loss of body function, divorce, and any number of significant factors can lead to chronic pain problem. Nonetheless, pain is just pain. Generally it's nothing life-threatening, unless one uses narcotics, injections, or surgery. Certainly occasional suicides occur, but these are rarely seen in people employing mind-body techniques. Suicides occur when patients are addicted to drugs. I know of no one in our holistic pain clinics who have committed suicide, but I personally know a number who committed suicide following narcotic prescriptions, overdosing, and unnecessary usage.

Pain means different things to different people. Some cultures barely believe in it. I know an Amish man who had his arm literally in the air in a cast for months; I asked him if he had any pain, and he said he was too busy to think of it. He runs a furniture factory and had a serious electrical injury. To top it all off, this was neuropathic pain. So the human mind is greatly involved in pain problems. The pain certainly is real to the patient; I never doubt it or suggested that it is not. Whether there is a clear cause or not, the pain is real and must be treated. It could be formed or changed brain chemistry.

Hospitals, emergency rooms, and pain clinics all over the country, medical providers and manufacturing companies, especially pharmaceutical companies, are making a fortune from the unclear diagnosis of these chronic pain patients. The treatment with addictive medications aggravates the situation greatly, and so are many injections and surgeries. Look at the websites of many pain centers—I see little evidence of a holistic approach. The insurance companies also should be criticized for not paying for holistic approaches. I told an insurance executive the other day that they should reduce the payments for narcotic prescriptions. He was not interested. We all criticize the food industry for giving us bad food, but believe me, if we requested good food, they would be providing it—they like to make money. It's no different for the pain industry. If they would stop paying for excessive narcotic use, the providers would not be giving it, and they would demand cash up front before they wrote the script. Many people are collecting disability payments based on pain. Ten million are on Social Security disability, and probably fifty percent of them could work. How do I know that? I've worked with them every day and have for forty-one years. Work can distract from pain and could have great value. But who can read the human mind? The economy is poor; people need to survive. *I can't find a job, but maybe I can collect disability to pay the bills.* I see that daily. It's impossible to criticize that, but we know what it is: dishonesty. Lawyers make a lot of money from fraudulent lawsuits. Who's involved? Lawyers, patients, and medical providers. I've seen it for years. It's actually a fraud, is it not? Social security doesn't pay when it should, yet to the pain clinic they pay too easily.

Pain may be one of our senses, like hearing, touching or seeing. Aristotle said pain is an emotion, like laughter or joy. Fear of pain can be worse than the pain itself. The waterboarding methods used by the military to get information out of terrorists proved that fear of the act is worse than the act itself. Asian cultures think pain is due to excessive energy or chi. Acupuncture moves chi to another part of the body.

Metabolic Pain

Chronic pain without clear cause is a serious national problem. Many of these patients are dependent or addicted to narcotics or other serious medication. Remember, acute pain tells you what the problem is, you correct the problem, and the pain is gone. There is no addiction to pain medication unless the provider has not established an endpoint to the prescription. Acute pain accounts for about ten percent of the pain problems. Another ten percent or so is chronic neuropathic pain, the pain associated with nerve damage, an amputated extremity, diabetic neuropathy, or a pinched nerve. These patients sometimes need narcotic medication for short- or long-term relief. Then again, if you apply the 30/30 rule, narcotics don't help that much and patients run the risk of addiction. Also remember that anyone can get addicted to a drug in a week, cigarettes sometimes within a day. That tells you the danger of using medications when they are not needed. Long-term use of medications, especially narcotics, can result in "sensitization," when you become much more sensitive to light pain stimuli, and "allodynia," in which the threshold of pain appreciation has changed. If you touch the skin of a person addicted to narcotics for chronic pain, they may be extremely sensitive. With increasing usage of narcotics, a person becomes tolerant, his neurotransmitters change, and he constantly needs an increasing dose of medication because of this tolerance and change in brain chemistry. The whole body has become sensitized, and the pain threshold has changed. Tolerance leads to habituation, which leads to addiction. Addiction is characterized by overwhelming craving and willingness to do unreasonable things to get the medicine. What about the other sixty to seventy percent of the nonneuropathic pain people? Some have conditions like nociceptive pain, osteoarthritis, rheumatoid arthritis, tennis elbow, or bursitis. The people with nociceptive pain represent maybe ten percent of the pain problem. The rest are without clear cause and account for a huge number, and are at a very serious risk for addiction to narcotics. We don't even know why they hurt. The patients with nociceptive pain can generally be treated physically, with a minimum of pain medication, and the great majority don't need narcotic medication. Even if they say their pain is 9 on a scale of 1 to 10, doctors should resist the use of narcotics because of the risk of addiction, habituation and sensitization. Once a person becomes addicted, they are considered to be an addict the rest of their lives according to most psychiatrists, even if they are not taking the medication. You can see the seriousness of the problem. So what do we call that forty percent or so (some think its 50-90%) who have chronic pain without a clear cause? Chronic pain books don't even have a suggestion or name for this percentage of people with chronic pain. Since they are the ones more likely to become addicted because their pain is most likely based on the chemistry of the brain, we desperately need to change this. I like the term "Metabolic Pain (centralized brain pain) because it's not insulting; it doesn't imply that pain is in the patient's head or due to a chemical. I ran this name past an excellent psychiatrist who deals a lot with pain and addiction to pain medication on a daily basis, and he thinks that's a good pick. Actual chemicals, neuropeptides, hormones, and neurotransmitters are activated by our thought processes, affect the rest of the body, and can cause pain, mostly originating in the metabolic center of the hypothalamus. The brain speaks to the body through neurotransmitters and neuropeptides. Diagnostic tests find nothing. Our autonomic nervous system, the sympathetic and parasympathetic, can also cause pain through neurotransmitters and nerve-impulse conduction. Hopelessness, anger, anxiety, and depression affect chemistry of the brain only and yet can produce a state of pain in the body. Many people have been addicted to habituated medications and narcotics. These patients are the heart of the pain centers. Many may be masquerading with a nocebo diagnosis, one based on a CT, MRI, or angiogram that has nothing to do with their medical problem. This is the excuse a lot of pain centers use to overtreat these patients. It also gives centers a method of billing for their injections and giving narcotics. I've seen some pain centers inject a hundred people a day.

What is a good definition of addiction? The World Health Organization likes to use the word dependency, physical and mental, and drop the word addiction. Others disagree. Addiction and habituation combine mental and physical dependency, compulsive behavior that harms a person. A person is addicted when they can no longer keep out of harm's way. Addiction causes a change in the chemistry of the brain. When the change occurs, people lose control over their own urges. They are so compelled that nothing else matters. It does not matter how intelligent a person is, these impulses can affect all of us. Dependency is one step along the path. One day the switch is thrown to addiction. It can occur in a day, a week, a month, or a year; it's very unpredictable. Once you are addicted, psychiatrists say you are addicted for life, even if you are not taking the addictive substance. You can return to becoming addicted in a minute. Addiction is a chronic and dangerous disease, so avoidance is critical. Don't take that narcotic medication unless you have acute or neuropathic pain. Unless there is clear cause, you don't take it more than once or twice a week.

Addiction takes many forms—medication, illegal drugs, sex, cigarettes, alcohol, etc. It devastates families, destroys health and jobs, and many lead to death—seventy in my area this year, fifteen thousand in the nation. It is a psychological disorder, a family dysfunction, a physical need. Addiction is a combination of mental and physical attendance. Mental dependence refers to one's mind because specific events trigger emotional and physical urges. Memory circuits set off by various stimuli produce a series of chain reactions producing biochemically urgent, overwhelming cravings.

There's a difference between physical and mental dependence. Mental dependence develops by changes in chemistry brought on by the thought process. Thinking changes brain chemistry and the chemistry of one's mind-body, body-mind. Physical dependence involving no thinking reflects the physical effects of the addictive substance on one's neurotransmitters. When people gain tolerance, that's a physical effect. Their neurotransmitters change. Chronic pain is a disease of the CNS that may or may not correlate with any tissue damage. The neural circuits have changed. Just narcotics could do it over a short period of time. They may convert acute, neuropathic, or metabolic Pain (centralized brain pain) into another disease, chronic pain, and addiction.

The fifty percent or so of chronic pain patients whom I like to call "chronic metabolic Pain (centralized brain pain) patients" are products of overprescribed narcotic medication, yet in most pain books they don't have a name. Some say they suffer from idiopathic pain, but who wants to be an idiot, or pathetic? So I like the name metabolic Pain (centralized brain pain). We just keep on giving these chronic metabolic pain patients another prescription or do a procedure on them. Even psychiatrists like the term metabolic Pain (centralized brain pain). Patients don't like to hear that pain is in their heads, that they have a mental problem, or that the doctor doesn't know why they hurt. They may believe the doctor thinks it's in their head or they are making it up.

Another significant problem is patients who need the diagnosis of pain to get a disability check. Yes, this is a reality. Probably fifty percent of people on Social Security disability carry a pain diagnosis. No pain, no check. You can imagine the economic impact of that, especially when they're receiving disability checks for many years. When they're better they are supposed to go to Social Security and tell them they're well, but don't hold your breath. Only three percent of the patients on Social Security disability ever return to work. This has great economic and psychological impact on the patient.

The point is, providers should at least have the decency not to give patients narcotics just because they feel sorry for their economic situation. This is also a very common problem in the Veterans Administration system. A lot of long-term disability is dependent on "I hurt." The nocebo or negative talk of diagnostic tests is used commonly to get disability. This type of pain, I think, is chemically based—neurotransmitters, lack of serotonin, lack of dopamine, hopelessness, anxiety, depression, and economic need. The electrophysiology and biochemistry of the brain and body, the psychology, produced this perception of pain, consciously or subconsciously. We consider the pain to be real. But the doctor must be alert. The word of the patient is not the gold standard; the diagnosis is the gold standard. To be frank, you can't just say "I believe you" to everyone. Doctors must be alert, otherwise they will addict the whole town, and believe me, I am witnessing it. We have a national scandal going on. It involves the providers, patients, industrial and pharmacological industry, and emergency rooms and hospitals, especially radiologists who overuse x-rays to provide an excuse for overtreating the patient.

Pain is a complex and active network that involves many brain modules. Psychiatric pain syndromes can involve the autonomic nervous system, sympathetic and parasympathetic; the CNS, with the production of neuropeptides, hormones, and neurotransmitters; the limbic system; hypothalamus; and yes, even the immune system. All the neuropeptides made by the brain also are made by the white cells of the blood, the immune system. Mind-body, body-mind. Because of that, the rest of the body also can be involved—the heart, gastrointestinal system, skin, spine, muscles, etc. The whole body can become sensitized to narcotic medication.

There's no reason to hand out narcotics for metabolic or idiopathic pain, or pain with no clear cause, as it surely will habituate or addict the patient eventually. Because of tolerance, the development of sensitization, people will continue to need to increase medication. I see it on a daily basis. The pain centers are having a ball with it. It's a spinning wheel that never ends, and it ruins many lives. I see it all the time.

ADDICTED INFANTS

The number of infants addicted through their mothers has tripled in ten years. As if you could not guess! Yes, many physicians' prescriptions have addicted the mothers. It's occurring all over the country. The prescriptions are not given for very good reasons. An excellent study came out of the University of Michigan and was published in the *Journal of the American Medical Association* recently. Around three and a half percent of babies born in hospitals in 2009 all over the country had drug withdrawal at birth because their mothers were habituated or addicted when the infant was in the womb. The international definition of addiction has now dropped the word "addiction" and just uses the term "habituation and dependency" Usually illegal behavior is part of the definition of addiction, which of course is not possible for a newborn. The World Health Organization changed the definition. The infants have withdrawal symptoms, irritability, difficulty breathing, low birth weight, feeding problems, and they cry a lot. Some even die. These problems generally involve very long hospitalizations, and over ninety percent of the time, Medicaid pays for it . The cost is estimated at $700 million at this time, and soon it will be $1 billion, as the problem is not going away and actually is increasing. These infants are the most vulnerable members of society. Mothers of course should not be taking any opiate or opioid medications during pregnancy. But let me tell you, it's difficult for a habituated or addicted person to make such a decision. The brain is so focused on getting the high or getting back to basic normal that the brain is hardly functional, and it's near impossible to make a good decision. You can blame them all you want but I'm familiar with these patients. Most of them are started on a narcotic prescription given for non-malignant pain problems, "metabilic pain (centralized brain pain)." That's where the real mistake is. Many of these young mothers are under horrible, psychological, social, and economic stress, and a significant number of these pregnancies were unexpected. Many of these women are not married, and many do not have family support to get the dopamine and serotonin to make it through the day, which is unfortunately quite common. A national scientific study by Dr. Stephen Patrick, a neonatologist from the University of Michigan, found that it is the epidemic of the providers' drug prescriptions that is doing it. About four and a half percent of pregnant women are using illegal drugs according to the CDC. But I say they are wrong—it's the "legal addict," the woman with the script provided by a doctor. Usually the newborn is given a methadone oral spray to reduce the withdrawal symptoms, and the mother is placed on an oral methadone. Methadone is an opioid and actually dangerous to use, although they have to use it. It has a long half-life and can cause cardiac arrhythmias resulting in death. There was a cardiac arrest in my hospital just recently—the patient was on methadone and had no evidence of heart disease.

Newborns who have opioid withdrawal are generally small and at high risk of death. Many end up with neurological health problems as adults. Nurses and doctors can tell which babies are going through withdrawal by their cries, diarrhea, and failure to grow. You would think this would stimulate the government agencies and medical societies to reeducate the medical community as to what the appropriate treatment of pain is, instead of starting this addictive process with prescriptions. The problem is huge! Don't expect the pain societies to lead the way. A Medicaid fraud unit could do it. Let's face it, Medicaid is part of this because they are paying the bill. They even paid the taxi driver to take the addicted patient to their medical provider for a refill. They pay the taxi driver, the pain center, and the narcotic provider, they pay for the medicine, and then they pay for the horrible complications habituation leads to. The Medicaid fraud unit needs to step up to bat.

Weaning infants from drugs can take months and is extremely expensive but it needs to be done. I've confirmed that myself by speaking to the neonatologist at a hospital. This person even told me the name of a town where a lot of these infants come from. The incidence of this is growing by leaps and bounds. These addicted newborns have been more commonly found in Maine, Florida, Georgia, West Virginia, Kentucky, and other parts of the Midwest according to Dr. Stephen Patrick's article in *U.S. News and World Report*, from which I am liberally quoting.

* * *

The Struggle

August, 2010

(The names of the physicians mentioned in the following story have been changed in order to protect their identity. This is the patient's story in her own words.)

I went into the bathroom. Got the Opana out of the bottle. Cut it up into fine powder. Used an empty pen and snorted it into my nose. It was time for bed so I took my trazodone for sleep and my Chantex. Crawled under the covers. I remember feeling like I could leave my body. I went to sleep. I dreamt that I was at the top of a staircase.

Everything was so dark. Somebody pushed me from behind, I thought.

"Mrs. James, we are putting you into a CT scan" were the first words I heard that morning. I was at the emergency room and it was explained to me that my husband heard me scream and found me in a pool of blood coming from my head. I had fallen down our staircase. My bedroom is situated upstairs.

I had cracked my head wide open on the tile floor, fractured my scapula, put my knee through the drywall toward the end of the staircase.

I waited as they stapled my head together, put my arm in a sling, and of course they asked if I had pain medicine. I told them that I did. My back and my body hurt like hell.

At that time, I wondered why I didn't die. Why didn't God just relieve all the pain I was in.

I felt enough was enough! I was a captive to the pain pills. I was on Opana 40 mg 4 x a day for severe back pain. My tolerance was now so high that I was abusing it. I was snorting the medicine. I couldn't stop. I ran out of medicine two weeks before I should have. I would go through severe withdrawal until I picked up my next prescription. I would buy medicine from anyone who had it. Then start withdrawal all over again. There was no hope left.

From Narcotics Anonymous book, 6th Edition:

"For us, using became a habit and finally was necessary for survival. The progression of the disease was not apparent to us. We continued on the path of destruction unaware of where it was leading us. We were addicts and did not know it."

I was slowly committing suicide.

* * *

The Accident

June, 2000

I hurt my back by lifting too much weight. I did some landscaping and worked at a home improvement store here in town. I worked in the garden department and went to help someone in the cabinet department. I lifted, pulled, and pushed over fifty cabinets and I felt something happen to my back.

I remember lying in my bed rolled into a ball crying. My lower spine and buttocks were in pain and just wouldn't stop. It never did.

The first doctor I went to really didn't know what was wrong with me. He did not do any x-rays or tests. He wrote me a prescription for Vicodin. I had never been on pain medicine before.

The Vicodin made me feel great. I could run all over work and do my job. There was very little pain and it made me very hyper. After a while the Vicodin stopped working. The pain became unbearable and eventually I had to quit my job because it was very physical. I was taking more and more Vicodin.

I went to an orthopedic doctor who did some x-rays. He informed me that I had pulled my right side pelvis back and down. He told me I needed physical therapy.

I went to physical therapy for a while but the physical therapist just couldn't get the spasms or the pain to slow down. I ended up at my first pain doctor.

They told me that the pain pills would give me a better quality of life. What they didn't tell me was that this kind of life led to death.

* * *

The Doctors

Dr. Garcia put me on Fentanyl patches. They didn't work very well. I heard weird noises in my head. He did some procedures on my back.

They made the pain worse. I had an argument with his nurse over the phone. She said they were going to increase my medicine to morphine and that I had to take it. I said, "No I'm not." She said, "Yes you are." She continued to tell me that I had to take it. I refused. I was so angry I gave the phone to my husband.

A couple of days later I received a letter in the mail stating that Dr. Garcia's office would not see me anymore. I had to find another pain doctor before I ran out of my medicine.

I was going to Dr. Smithers. He was my family doctor. I remember screaming in his office as he did procedures on me. He put needles in my muscles and broke them up. He was the one who sent me to "the god."

Dr. Marley had a very impressive title on his door. Surely this man could help me. If I had only known. I can remember some of the things he did to me. Most of it now in my memory is wrapped in darkness.

Dr. Marley did an MRI. They didn't find anything. But I was still living in the spasms and pain. Dr. Marley put me on OxyContin. His nurse said I could have a choice of three drugs: OxyContin, methadone, or morphine. Actually giving you a choice! Looking back, I can't believe they can get away with that! I knew morphine (from an experience in the hospital) gave me hallucinations, I knew methadone was for heroin addicts, so I said OxyContin. I didn't know anything about it except I'd heard it helped pain. I chose the drug from hell. My descent into addiction to prescription pain pills really began.

Dr. Marley did every procedure on my back he could possibly do. Epidurals, nerve blocks, burning the nerves in my back. With each one my pain got worse. They never helped. My OxyContin intake increased They added other narcotics like Vicodin, Percocet, and oxycodone for the breakthrough pain. I was put on sleep meds also. I remember having a storage bag full of drugs. By that time I was in my ghost-like state. I didn't even know what they were doing to me. I just wanted to be able to get out of bed. I wanted the spasming and the pain in my glutes and back to stop. It would only get worse.

By then my son started to steal my medicine. He stole my OxyContin. I called Dr. Marley's office and told them what had happened. They told me to come in to the office. I took my husband in with me. They said they couldn't help me anymore.

* * *

PAIN

Dr. Ted (the Arrogant)

At first I thought Dr. T was a pleasant sort of fellow. He immediately put me on more meds. I thought he understood how I felt. More MRIs showed nothing wrong with me. My spine looked fine. But immediately he wanted to do injections—SI joint injections, facet injections, epidurals, etc.

I wasn't making good choices. I was not in my right mind at all due to the narcotics. He seemed adamant about doing them. So one by one the injections were done, each one bringing with it more pain. Only after lying in bed for days, I finally would calm down some.

I remember at some point being on a narcotic called Kadian. It was getting slowly increased over time. Of course I was on the regular breakthrough narcotics to help also with the pain. I was on all these pain medications. I lay in bed most of the day, barely getting my husband dinner. When they increased the narcotics, I would feel a little better. I could do things around the house but my tolerance was getting higher. They didn't work for very long.

My son was stealing my pain medicines. I remember having an electronic safe. He even broke his way into that. That would throw me into withdrawl because I would be short on my medication. The withdrawl would make me wish for death. It was unbearable.

I was in and out of St. Joe Hospital trying to get off the pain medications but I would end up back on them because I could not take the pain.

For years I was in this cycle. I remember seeing a Dr. Fowler, a well-known back surgeon at an orthopedic center here in town. He said he couldn't help me, but of course directed me to their pain physicians, who prescribed more narcotics and did trigger-point injections. One of the ortho pain doctors stood out in my mind.

* * *

Dr. Adams

I had been off pain meds for about three months but I could barely endure the pain. I was ending up at the emergency room too many times. They knew who I was. They kept referring me back to pain doctors.

Dr. Adams said he was going to put me back on OxyContin. I stood in that little room and cried.

Dr. Adams wanted to do a new procedure on me that he said could help the pain. He said it could be done in Warsaw, Indiana, where they have resuscitation machinery. He wanted to run anesthesia through my veins. I thought this is something new so I said yes. I met them in Warsaw where they hooked up the IV. He ran the anesthesia. I felt okay on the ride home because he had given me another medicine through the IV that made you feel good.

That evening I started feeling like a man was sitting on my chest. My chest hurt bad. I still felt that way the following morning. I called the ortho place where Dr. Adams worked. They told me to call an ambulance right away. So I dialed 911.

My blood pressure was sky high. One of the ambulance workers put nitrates under my tongue. I felt this horrible headache come on fast. They said it was from the nitrates. Once again I was at the emergency room. The nurse hooked me up to an EKG. My head was okay. After seeing the doctor I was released.

I told Dr. Adams I wanted an EMG, which came back showing an abnormal L4-L5 level. After that was a discogram which showed that L5-S1 looked shattered. I couldn't believe it. All this time with the MRI, and only the discogram had found it.

I was set up to see an orthopedic surgeon. Dr. Smith and I both thought surgery would be a good option. All this time and now we found it.

I would get better, or so I thought.

I now realize that I was not in my right mind. I was in my ghostly haze making decisions all alone. I was so screwed up on the drugs.

After surgery they had me on a drip for pain, but after I went home I was in tremendous pain.

The surgery made me very weak. The pain moved from my hips, my back felt crushed. I felt very weird nerve pain crawling and pricking all around my hips, back, and buttocks. My feet felt like I was walking on crushed glass.

I went to physical therapy at a very good place here in town. We did aquatic therapy in a very warm pool. While I was on my pain meds, everything was as good as could be expected. Then I decided once again to come off my pain meds. I packed a suitcase and checked myself into a local hospital.

I crammed myself in a bed. I remember the pain was so bad I could hardly walk. I can't explain withdrawl—sweats, cold, a dirty feeling, vivid nightmares, and dreams so real you feel that they really happened. You feel so much pain you want to die so it will end.

When my husband came to pick me up from the hospital I was in so much pain I could barely walk. Remember, this was right after surgery. I remember sitting in our living room chair. All I could do was sit in the chair or lie down. I thought I was crazy for coming off the medicine so fast after surgery. I was thinking, "I can't live like this."

I contacted an acute pain doctor's office. I couldn't believe it. He was going to see me! He put me on a drug called Opana. It worked pretty well. I could do some things again! Go to grocery store, make my husband's dinner, normal things, etc. I did not know at the time that Opana at some point turns on you. And after a while it did.

Through time the Opana stopped working. All I did was lie in bed. I was so tired all the time. When I slept was the only time the pain was gone. I could get some relief from my suffering.

The doctor's NP continued to up my dose until I was finally on the highest dose of medicine (Opana) that there was.

It worked for a while and then it wasn't working so well. My son said, "Mom, let me show you how to snort the medicine. It works a lot faster and better." I was truly out of my mind. I was so doped up I said okay, I'll try it.

It worked really well. I felt much better. I didn't realize it was the end of all the pain pills I had.

I had no relationships with my family, my God, my spirit and soul—all my creativity was taken away from me all those years. But I did not realize what the narcotics had done to me. They had shut my feelings down. I wasn't Pam anymore. I was a ghost in my body.

I was going through my medicine so fast that summer 2010. It was gone within two weeks. The withdrawl was so bad it took me about four days to get out of bed to take a shower. I lay in my bed writhing in pain praying to die. I could not stop it. I was a slave to the drug Opana.

I would buy more medicine from a lady who had a script for Opana. She would lie to the doctor and get Opana and sell each pill for $40 apiece. One pill would last for about six hours at the most, and then I would go back into withdrawal.

The doctor (Dr. Burke) could not get me on any narcotic that was higher in dosage because I was on the highest dose I could be on. My tolerance to drugs was so high that nothing worked anymore. I was at the lowest point of my life.

I started taking Chantex to quit smoking. I think the mixture of the drugs is why I sleepwalked the night I fell down the stairs.

* * *

2 Samuel 22

"The grave wrapped its ropes around me; death itself stared me in the face. But in my distress, I cried out to the Lord. He heard me from his sanctuary; my cry reached His ears."

After I fell down the stairs in August of 2010, I knew I was going to die. Two months later, I called my mother. She lives in Hudson, IN. I told her that I was going to die and that I needed help. She told me that she was living in fear of a phone call at night saying that I was dead. But she and her friend had been praying and praying through all these years. They never gave up.

At that point, I really know that God took over. Two days later I was on a plane to Palm Beach to detox at a place called the Summerhouse. The place is run by long-term recovering addicts. It was a nice place. They detoxed us so slowly you could barely tell you were detoxing. I had two roommates, both young girls addicted to prescription drugs. One was addicted to Xanax, the other to "blues." So sad. Everyone in the placed seemed to be addicted prescription narcotics. It was mostly young adults.

I had a nurse who checked blood, checked vitals, and handed me my medicine for withdrawal. Thank God my liver and kidneys results came back fine.

We had a chef who cooked our meals. My room had a big fluffy bed with a white comforter on it. I had a flat-screen TV and two nice roommates.

At lunchtime, the iguanas came out to sun themselves. We were situated on a canal. I would sit and watch the water sparkle and the parakeets fly overhead. I was a million miles away from home.

* * *

Rehab: The Orchid

Arriving at the Orchid, I was not doing too well. The narcotics were out of my system. The pain felt raw, more intense. I was not happy to hear the rule about no telephone for two weeks, then only two ten-minute telephone calls on Saturday and Sunday.

The learning center was a few miles away from our living quarters. We were usually at the learning center. We never had a chance to breathe. When I arrived, they went through all my luggage. I was pissed. I was in pain. My mood was not pretty. They immediately took me to a room where everyone was playing a game. It was called a fun day. I sat down in a chair and said, "Ten thousand dollars to play a f—ing game!" Everyone looked at me but just continued playing. I sat there broiling!

We finally went a couple miles away to where we stayed; it was beautiful. This place was also run by long-term recovering addicts, very intelligent women. You could also tell it was decorated by women. I had a nice bedroom. But I was still not happy. I was in pain.

The night sweats continued. Bad vivid dreams. They just wouldn't stop. I had post-acute withdrawal syndrome. I had never heard of that, but it was one of the many things I would learn. One of the first things I was to learn was they were not going to put up with my bitching about my pain. I was expected to do almost everything anyone did.

The schedule here was rigid; you woke up here by 7:00 and had to be ready to go by 8:00. I usually woke up around 4:00 to read my Bible and to have a quiet time before the day began. Then breakfast, make beds, all dishes done, and that bed better be made right or you had to remake it. I remember this with a fondness now, but at the time I thought it was like boot camp!

We learned about the disease of addiction, we learned about our emotions, feelings which had been arrested by our disease. We learned how to get them out. There were creative arts. We went to a museum in Palm Beach. I had never seen anything like the art I saw there.

We went to a labyrinth in a church. I learned about my drug-seeking behavior and how it worked. We had a therapist who worked with us one on one about once a week and handed out all the assignments to do. I had a few on chronic pain. I can't believe I did it with the way I felt. My back felt crushed.

When we arrived back at our rooms we made dinner and cleaned up, and then every night we attended meetinga—AA, NA, and CA meetings. I really liked the meetings. They are the thing to keep you off the drugs.

Most of all I learned who I was: a creative, loving, and compassionate woman, and I had many blessings in my life. I made some friends who I know will be lifelong. That was such a blessing also.

I was shaky; I was also suffering from post-acute withdrawal. I felt sometimes like I could just break, but I was alive and narcotic-free when I arrived home just before Christmas.

I started attending Narcotics Anonymous meetings the next day. I started Intensive Outpatient (IOP) at St. Joe Hospital. I put everything I had into it. I continued to learn about the disease of addiction and more about myself.

After a couple of months the women at IOP wanted me to see a pain doctor named Dr. Womack. At first I refused but then gave in because I needed someone to give me my nonnarcotic medicine.

When I went in to see Dr. Womack I told her, "No narcotics and I mean it." She kept me on my Lyrica and muscle relaxers. That was the worst I have seen as far as a doctor using patients for money. As I had to wait in her office, I talked to people. I met people who were just in her office to get their narcotic scripts and go out to sell them. One young man told me that his cousin was going to be at Dr. Womack's office later that day to pick up her scripts because she sold them. One guy was so messed up on drugs he could barely walk, and he was going to drive home! I wish I had been a news reporter!

Dr. Womack's office was packed wall to wall with people. She wouldn't give anyone a script if they owed her money. I really saw a money-hungry doctor. She knew what she was doing. I finally had enough. I couldn't stand to see what was going on in that office.

I told my family doctor that I refused to go back. I told her that I felt like I was living in a drug house. She said she would take over the scripts so I would not have to go back there.

It has now been one year and three months that I have been narcotic-free. I attend Narcotics Anonymous meetings every week. I have a home group with people that really impact my life. I love them dearly. I am blessed with my husband. We have been married twenty-five years. He stayed with me through all the ugliness. He is a rock. I have earned all his trust back. I have a beautiful grandson. My son is now in recovery. I am back with family (mom, brothers, sister, etc.) mentally and spiritually. I love God with all my heart. I am truly a very blessed woman.

Yes, I still live in pain. I manage to deal with it on a daily basis. One day at a time.

I believe I have good, caring doctors. Every doctor I see I tell them, "I'm an addict." I firmly tell them, "No narcotics."

I take time every day for my devotions and time with God as I understand him.

I guess if I could just help anyone who is going through or is just coming out of addiction like what I went through these last ten years, it would be worth it to me. I pray that God uses me to help and minister to others. To give back what I have been given—the grace that God and family and others have given me.

1 John 5

God is light and there is no darkness in Him at all.

Psalm 116

I love the Lord because he hears and answers my prayers. Because he bends down and listens I will pray as long as I have breath! Death had its hands around my throat; the terrors of the grave overtook me. I saw only trouble and sorrow. Then I called on the name of the Lord; please, Lord, save me!

How kind the Lord is! How good he is!

So merciful this God of ours!

The Lord protects those of childlike faith; I was facing death, and then he saved me.

Now I can rest again,

for the Lord has been so good to me.

He has saved me from death,

my eyes from tears

my feet from stumbling,

And so I walk in the Lord's presence

as I live here on earth!

I believe in you!

(This is the patient's story in her own words)

* * *

Cathy's Story

I am not sure where to begin my story as there is so much to tell. I am currently thirty-six. I am an educated individual who attended nursing school back in the 90s and I am now currently in school studying law and criminal justice. I am one of the unfortunate people who is currently unemployed, without health insurance. I rely on free health clinics and hospitals for my medical care and my prescriptions.

I will start with my most recent visit to the clinic and emergency room. I had a sinus infection so I tried to get into the health clinic. I was unable to do so, so my only other choice to get antibiotics was to go to the emergency room and seek treatment. I went to one of the local emergency rooms that I have frequented the past two years. I told the doctor I had a sinus infection—green mucus, sinus congestion, facial pain. After a very short exam I was given ibuprofen to help ease my pain. The physician on duty deemed I did in fact have a sinus infection. He wrote me a script for antibiotics and then asked if I wanted something for pain. My friend who was with me recorded the conversation on her phone because I knew walking into the ER that I would be offered pain meds. The doctor and I discussed what antibiotics I would be put on as I had just been treated for a sinus infection the month prior. Then we discussed what I could get for my facial pressure and pain. Here is the actual recorded conversation:

Dr: "Do you need something stronger at home for pain just in case too?"
Me: "Um, no, I should be okay."
Dr: "You feel okay with ibuprofen or Tylenol? Either way. Okay, so if—okay, so if you got enough headache we can give ya a little Darvocet or something if you've had something like that before. If you don't want it that's okay."
Me: "Okay."
Dr: "I won't twist your arm."
Me: "No, it will probably help."

PAIN

Dr: "Have you had Darvocet before? It didn't make you sick or nauseous? Okay, let's give you a dose of ibuprofen, and give ya a script for Darvocet and a script for doxycycline."

I was released from the emergency room with my prescription for an antibiotic and for Darvocet. See actual script:

WARNING: THE FACE OF THIS DOCUMENT HAS A COLORED SECURITY PANTOGRAPH BACKGROUND ON WHITE

CATHY A. HAYNES

NAME: 14323 HAND RD FORT WAYNE, IN 46818   9/23/2010

DDRESS: Acct# 9023924   SSec#   DATE:

RX: Darvocet N-100   ☐ 1-24
QTY: 15   ☐ 25-49
SIG: 1 Q 4 Hrs   ☐ 50-74
PRN Pain   ☐ 75-100
          ☐ 101-150
No refills
Refill NR 1 2 3 4 5 VOID After ___   ☐ 151 and

___ M.D.   ___
Dispense as Written   May Substitute

This is truly how easy it is to get pain medicine from an emergency room. It is not just this one emergency room; it is all of them, and every single one I have been to.

When I first moved to Fort Wayne in 2008, I hurt my back moving. I went to a local emergency room (different than [the one I went to on] my most recent visit). As soon as I was taken to a room the nurses did an assessment and asked me what was wrong. I informed them I had hurt my back moving. I had low back pain, pain in my right buttock, and pain in my legs. The nurse put an IV in my arm and gave me a dose of morphine. The doctor came in and talked to me about my back and told me they would keep me for a little bit to help get my pain under control. About an hour later the nurse checked on me and I told her my pain was no better, so she gave me another dose of morphine. About fifteen minutes after that dose I began to break out in hives. I called the nurse in and they gave me a dose of Benadryl, and I informed her then that I was still in pain. A few minutes later she came back and gave me a dose of Dilaudid. Finally the pain subsided, somewhat. They sent me home with a prescription of Vicodin.

Between 2008 and to date I have been to the local emergency rooms for various reasons: cat bite, back injury or pain, body ache, upper respiratory infection, and so on. Every time I went to the emergency room I was given something for my pain: Dilaudid, Vicodin, Tylenol 3. I was given the pain medications via an injection or through an I.V. Always I was sent home with a script for either fifteen or thirty of the pain pills of choice.

In 1994 I had to have a right knee laparoscopy because I had a calcium buildup behind my kneecap. I remember coming out of surgery feeling like I flying: I was literally drooling on myself. I asked what they were giving me for the pain and they told me morphine. This was my first experience with morphine. It sure did ease the pain. I wanted more. After this particular surgery they sent me home with Percocet. I loved Percocet; it helped the pain and helped me sleep. I remember going through that prescription, and when I went back to the doctor for my post-op visit I asked for another prescription because I said my knee hurt so bad it was hard for me to sleep. I was handed a new script for thirty more Percocet without any questions.

May 2008 I had a total hysterectomy and bilateral oopherectomy. Prior to the surgery for about a month I was given all the pain pills I needed and asked for to keep me "comfortable" before my surgery. Of course, after my surgery I was given pain medicine and sent home with plenty as well.

Mother's Day of 2009 I was at the hospital visiting a friend. As I was leaving the hospital I subluxated my right hip. A nurse in the hallway helped me into a wheelchair and wheeled me over to the emergency room. A doctor came in asked me what happened and did an assessment. They hooked me up to an IV and were going to give me morphine. I told them that I was allergic to morphine due to my past reactions of breaking out in hives, and the fact that it just didn't work for me. They gave me Dilaudid. I was admitted to this particular hospital for four days. They had me hooked up to a machine that I could push the button when I needed pain medicine. The pain medicine I was given was Dilaudid. From my understanding and educational background, Dilaudid is pretty strong stuff. I know at one point of this stay I had so much pain medicine in my system I fell asleep with food hanging out of my mouth. One of my visiting friends thought this to be so funny they took pictures of it. There are some times of this stay I do not even remember because I was so drugged out. They took x-rays and could not find any damage from the injury. I was sent home with a prescription for pain medicine, again.

In May 2010 I was having colorectal issues and was scheduled for surgery in June. My doctor at the time gave me a prescription for pain medicine because of my complaint that it hurt when I had a bowel movement. Three weeks later when I had surgery, an anal ulcerectomy, I was sent home with another prescription for pain.

I don't remember the date; I can tell you that are were in 2009. I went to one of the local emergency rooms because my body just hurt. It was about a month or so before I was diagnosed with fibromyalgia. I went complaining of full-body pain and aches, nothing else. I was given Dilaudid via an injection and I believe some Toradol. I told the doctor they thought I had fibro but I had not yet been diagnosed. This doctor sent me home with Tylenol 3s.

I have been using pain pills since I was about fourteen, at least that is as far back as I can remember being prescribed pain pills. I have often wondered if my case is "one of a kind" when it comes to the ease of getting pain pills. At the age of fourteen my mother's chiropractor discovered I had spina bifida occulta. Since that point, getting pretty much any type of pain pill has been easy for me. There has <u>NEVER</u> been a time that I have requested pain pills and been denied. There are several times it has been offered without me asking. Even more, I can usually get my pain pill of choice. Again, I sit and think back, since I was fifteen, almost twenty years ago, I myself have had an open-ended availability of pain pills: Ultram, Percocet, Tylenol 3, Vicodin, Darvocet, morphine. You name it, I have had it.

If you go to my medicine box right this very moment, I have three different bottles of prescription pain pills: Vicodin, Darvocet, and Tylenol 3s. I keep them just in case I need them, yet I know that if I need more all I have to do is go to the emergency room.

As I sit here reading what I have written and looking back at all the pain medicine I myself have taken, I wonder how I never became addicted to pain pills. But then as I say that, I do realize that I have had my addiction to pain pills. For so long I could not sleep at night without taking at least two pain pills of choice and sometimes chasing it down with a Benadryl just so I could sleep. It was not until I was admitted to a psych ward for depression that the problem was brought to light. Part of my depression was caused by sleep problems and taking so much pain meds. I am lucky though because I was not what I would consider to be truly addicted. If you ask me now, though, to give you the three bottles of pain pills in my medicine box right now, I am not sure how easily I could give them to you. I live with pain; between my back and having fibromyalgia, I fear pain. I also wonder if my pain is caused by all the pain pills I have taken. My tolerance is so high now that nothing really does help but Dilaudid.

* * *

Working for Pain Management Doctors

It was about 1998 when I landed a job working for a group of pain management doctors in Indianapolis. Sadly my job only lasted about a month as I could not take the stress of working with doctors who deal with people who seek, who need, who had to have their pain meds.

I remember my first day as if it were yesterday. The office was chaotic and the phones rang and rang, never ending. The first phone call I ever took was an individual crying, begging for their pain medicine. I didn't know what to do. I took a message for the doctor as I normally would, only to have the patient call back four more times that day because they wanted their drug. Little did I know that first day how to me it would seem that those doctors approved the refills so easily.

By the second and third week I was shocked! The people coming into the office were lunatics—crazy fiends who wanted their drugs and would get them. Some patients would even be there waiting for you to harass you as you came or left the office. These people knew that their prescriptions could not be called in; they knew they had to have a written script. They knew what to say, they knew what to do. They knew even more than I did about some of the medicines they were seeking.

During visits some patients would cry, beg, and plead, telling you how much they needed their meds. Other patients would get angry and demand their pills. Some of these patients scared me. They knew that if a doctor denied them their drugs all they had to do was put up a fight and they got what they wanted. These people were on some serious pain medicines too. Some people had pain patches and took pain pills.

Working at this office was the first time I heard about the pain pill OxyContin. It seemed to me as if all the patients took this one particular pill. I felt as if we were giving out pain pills like they were candy; we were giving this candy to crazy people who sometimes scared me.

As I said, after about a month of freely passing out the pills and pain patches, I just could not take it anymore. I disagreed with it and I was scared by some of the patients as well. I had to give the job up.

* * *

My Best Friend's Mother

My best friend's mother—we will call her "C"—is the worst case scenario that I have seen of how easily these prescription drugs are given out and how easily they can ruin a life.

The first time I met C she was sitting in a chair with a walker in front of her. Her fingers were deformed and bent up due to arthritis. She seemed to me to be kind of "out of it," to describe her best. She was a very nice lady, but eventually I would see a different side of her.

After visiting with her a few times she pulled a large Ziploc bag out of the waistband of her pants. I was in awe and shock! Her little baggie had bottles—large bottles—of OxyContin, Percocet, and Vicodin. These were not your typical bottles with fifteen to thirty pills. I asked C what all the pills were for and she informed me they were all given to her for her pain. She told me that she was supposed to take the OxyContin every twelve hours and she did like clockwork, along with her other pain pills as well.

After about three of four months of knowing C, she called one day and requested we take her to the emergency room because "something was wrong." She told her daughter (my friend) and I that she didn't feel right and she needed to go to the emergency room. She moaned and groaned all the way there. Once inside the emergency room she said that she needed something for pain. She asked for morphine. As the nurse was out getting her choice of drug, C was in the room popping her OxyContin! After she was in the ER for about two hours, the doctor realized there was nothing he could find wrong with her, so he gave her a prescription for Vicodin and sent her on her way home.

It was about a month later when we went to visit C that she was crying because the pharmacy would not refill her OxyContin. They told her she had to wait one more day to get it filled. She was trembling and crying, stating that she felt as if she were going to die. It was a very scary sight to see.

Within in a few weeks we were making yet another trip to the emergency room. This time her mom claimed it was her head. Once we got to the ER it was the same old story and same old game. She got an IV with some pain meds in it, the doctors could find nothing wrong, and we were sent home with another prescription for pain pills.

About a month later, it was at the beginning of May 2009, her mom called crying about her leg. Apparently she had broken her tibia and she was in the hospital waiting for surgery the next day. We went to visit her that night in the hospital. Her mom seemed so out of it. You could tell she was "drugged." They had her on a pain pump and when the nurse went out of the room she was digging in her purse for her OxyContin. During her stay at the hospital she was on a morphine pain pump and taking Vicodin and OxyContin "on the side." I was in so much shock witnessing this: I just could not believe it.

After being released from the hospital for the surgery on her tibia, C had her OxyContin and her Vicodin. The doctor who gave her the Vicodin did not know about the OxyContin. She got her Vicodin filled and her OxyContin.

We went to visit her a few days later and she was almost out of both OxyContin and Vicodin. She was calling her doctor begging him for OxyContin. She still kept this baggie hidden in the waist of her pants, it had like three or four different bottles of pain meds. She always keeps it around her waist, so she always had it ready to go.

Literally a week later we were back at the emergency room because C was sure she had bronchitis or pneumonia. She was coughing horribly, which is to be expected because she smoked liked crazy. Her diet consisted of Coke, cigarettes, and pain pills. I only ever saw her eat two times in the three years I have known her. So here we go again. My roommate was at work so she asked me if I would take her mom [to the hospital], sure that she was truly sick. I on the other hand was skeptical as usual. I went to pick C up. She came out with her walker, her Coke, and a cigarette. She was coughing and hacking like you couldn't believe. I drove her to the emergency room, told them why we were there, and that we had just been there the week before, for "pain." They put us in a room and left us there for a bit. She talked and watched television. Finally they came to do x-rays on her chest. When they brought her back to the room she was moaning and groaning and complaining about how she couldn't take the pain, so of course they gave her more morphine. Once she had that, she was fine and ready to go home. The doctor said she had an upper respiratory infection and gave her some antibiotics—and, you guessed it, more Vicodin to take at home. When I called my roommate to let her know the story, she was so angry and upset. She was truly worried about her mom, and all her mom wanted was something to get her through the night so she could get her OxyContin filled the next day. Next day came and she got both her OxyContin and her Vicodin filled.

C, convinced that the doctors here in Fort Wayne were not good because they would only give her a script for OxyContin two times a day, decided to seek help outside the area. She contacted a doctor she had seen about fifteen years prior at the Cleveland Clinic in Cleveland, Ohio. This doctor is the doctor who had diagnosed her with rheumatoid arthritis so many years before. She just knew he would be the miracle she was seeking.

In the car we (my roommate, C, and I) went for a road trip to the Cleveland Clinic. We left early one morning because her appointment was at 1:45pm; it was a six-and-a-half hour drive from Fort Wayne. We made it there fifteen minutes late, but we did make it and the doctor was willing to see her being as how we had driven this far.

C was so happy to be able to see this doctor. She kept saying how he was a miracle worker and he would do something to help her pain. How he was the one who had diagnosed her when all other doctors told her she was crazy.

The doctor came in; he did not remember her, which instantly disappointed her. He inquired if she had been in physical therapy and what she was doing to help herself. Of course she could say nothing because all she had done was pop her pain pills, the pills which she was sure he would give her, only something better and more of it.

As the visit went on, it was clear the doctor was not a drug pusher like the ones back in Fort Wayne. He told her he wanted to do some x-rays and get a better picture of what was going on with her arthritis and the rest of her body. He ordered x-rays and blood work to be done.

By this time it was about four or five o'clock in the evening and we took C down to the first floor of the clinic to get her labs done. As she was being wheeled out from her labs she told the nurse she was having chest pain. This happened when she realized she was getting nothing from her "miracle" doctor that day other than the labs.

Of course the lab nurse took C seriously. She ran to get her some water and called 911. The next thing you know C was playing the nurse and the paramedics who came, telling them she was in pain and she would be okay but asking them if maybe she should go to the emergency room and get "something" just in case.

We followed through and got to the emergency room there at the Cleveland Clinic. Her mom was in a room complaining of pain and asking for pain meds. I took the ER doctor in the hallway and explained the whole long story to her—about how C was a drug seeker, was in the ER in Fort Wayne the week prior, and how she did not need pain medicine. The emergency room doctor told us she would not give C anything for pain but that she would assess all her other complaints.

When we went into the room to see C I told her that I had told the doctor she was a drug seeker and that the doctor would not be giving her any pain medicines. At this point C got very upset and was yelling at both me and my roommate (her daughter). Her daughter was so upset and distraught by the whole situation. Upset because at this point it was almost 9 p.m., we were in Cleveland, she had to be at work the next morning at 5 a.m., and her mom was begging for pain meds.

This situation in the emergency room in Cleveland went on for about two to three hours. Her mom, convinced that she should stay there and they would help finally, realizing she was going to get no pain pills, reluctantly stated she would go home.

The ride home was hell! Her mom was finally getting her own OxyContin out of her purse; coming down was a real bitch. She yelled, she sobbed, she fussed all the way home, telling her daughter how horrible she was and yelling at me because I was part of all this as well. She was so upset at us because she had gotten no more pain pills that night. C, who had us all convinced she needed help in and out of the car, hopped right out of the car on the way home when we got a flat so she could smoke. She did this with NO help, only the help of her pain pills.

After the Cleveland incident, which was about a year ago, neither I nor my roommate has spoken to or contacted C at all. She treated us so horribly, all because she could not get her pain pills that day from the doctor. I know that my roommate's other family members have kept in touch with C. They tell us she looks horrible. She can't think straight and she can't walk right. They say she still has her stash of meds and she is still getting the OxyContin. Sadly, she is losing her life, her family, and her friends, all to OxyContin and the doctors here who freely give them to her.

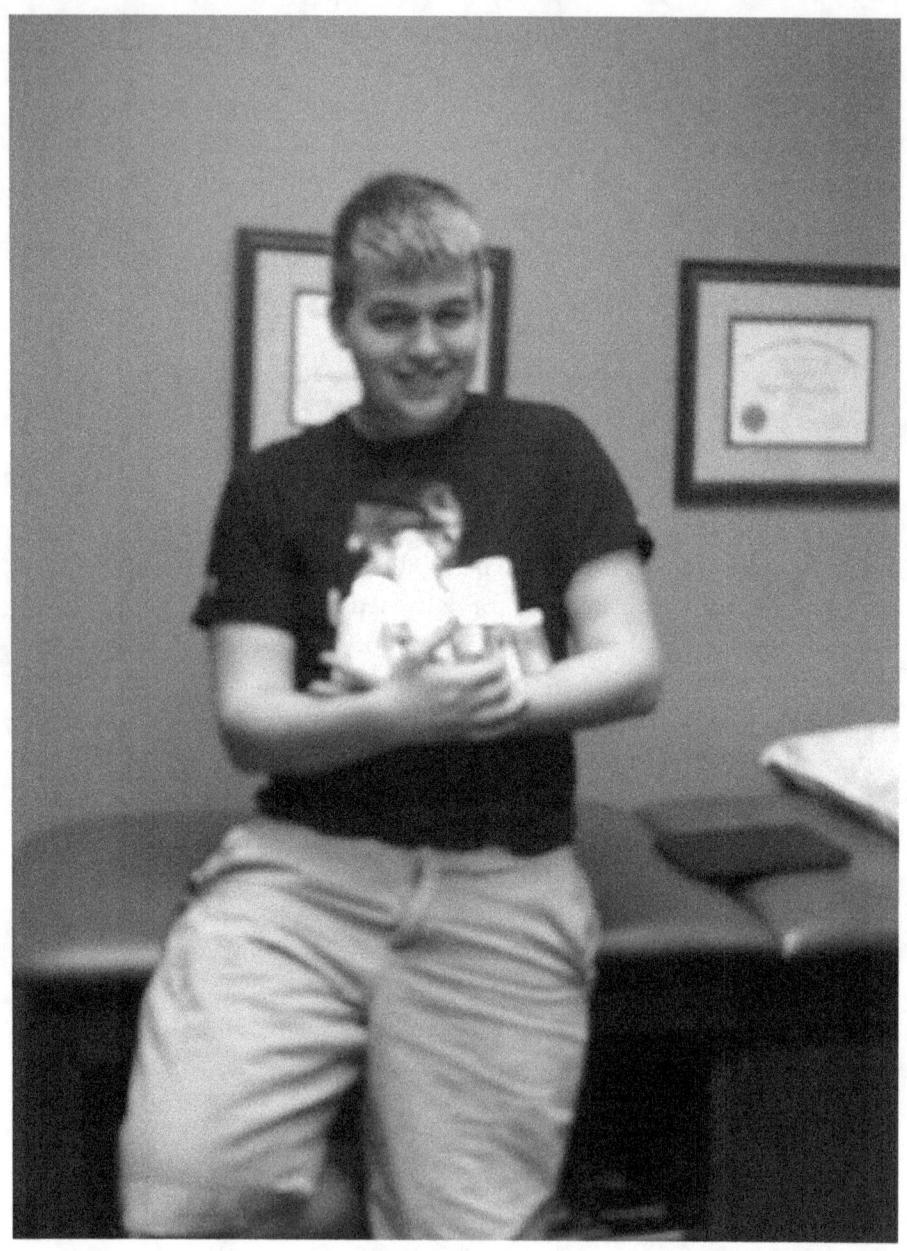

Erik Bailey, over treated by a Pain Center

PILL MILLS: A DANGER TO THE DESPERATE

by Erik Bailey High School Student

The ancient phrase "desperate times call for desperate measures" has never had greater meaning. The idea of experiencing constant, excruciating, and usually unexplained pain can make one jump at any opportunity to relieve their pain. These opportunities are when dangerous establishments titled "pill mills" decide to step in and order a solution that involves addiction, and sometimes death. Pill mills, also known as simply pain management clinics, can be found in every state, and in most towns. Such pain management clinics offer patients cheap, addictive, and effective drugs in order to create a stream of mindless consumers that arrive for an appointment every two months to hear a doctor promise that "they will soon be living free of medication." Unfortunately, after the doctor titters such a phrase, a prescription is then written to guarantee that the patient will arrive for the next appointment, where the same situation only repeats itself. One of the main reasons that such businesses are allowed to continue is due to both uneducated and ignorant landowners that allow them to practice on their property. Both small-time landowners and huge hospitals allow this dangerous consumer base to be produced on their land and are not aware of both the ethical and unlawful problems that can arise when these clinics are discovered.

Nearly fifty million Americans live with chronic pain every day. Not every pain management clinic prescribes medication. In fact, legitimate pain management clinics offer alternative plans such as exercise or diet changes, similar to physical therapy (WebMD). "These health care providers include doctors of different specialties as well as nonphysician providers specializing in the diagnosis and management of chronic pain" (WebMD.) Such nonphysician providers include acupuncturists and massage therapists. While it has been proven that clinics in these circumstances have been able to help their patients deal with the pain, these same clinics are able to prescribe addicting medication. These prescriptions can range from anything as mild as Tramadol, a mild pain killer, to an even more powerful opiate such as oxycodone (WebMD). Oxycodone exhibits side effects toward addiction similar to heroin. Even though pain management clinics are able to offer services not involving medication, many of them actually incorporate powerful medication immediately in order to ensure that they will be willing to return to the clinic. Patients are repeatedly told that they will soon be relieved of all medication, only to arrive two months later to hear the doctor utter the same words while handing them a piece of paper granting them relief until their next appointment. Such tactics from a business standpoint do make sense. The system allows doctors to easily trap patients in an endless cycle. While doing this, pain management doctors are able to maintain a steady income. Such business practices have been seen in retail stores across the world. The main difference is the use of such tactics in a medical office could potentially damage human life and comfort.

As pill mills across the United States have been discovered, they have in turn been shut down. The doctors in charge of such clinics are charged with second-degree murder and are sent to be tried in front of a judge. Some are sent to years of prison and are never able to practice medicine ever again in their life. In other cases some "doctors" that run the clinics actually do not hold a degree and are not supposed to be practicing medicine. Such people are openly deceiving their clients, and sometimes have resulted in their death. Recently, Florida shut down nearly thirteen "pill mills" and actually arrested and charged doctors with second-degree murder. Across these combined clinics, over thirty-two million pills of oxycodone have been prescribed to patients (Alvarez). In October of 2010, Florida introduced a ban on powerful pain pills limiting the amount that a doctor could prescribe (Alvarez). On the matter, Florida's Attorney General Pam Bondi stated, "We had no tough laws in place; now we do" (Alvarez). The same initiative needs to be taken across the United States in order to prevent more people being addicted to powerful opiates and to allow any potential death to be stopped. Every clinic in the United States that claims to be "pain management" needs to be investigated to ensure that alternative methods to deal with pain are taught to the patients rather than addictive medication which in turn will increase pain and bring their lives to a halt. In order for one to be cured of an oxycodone addiction, they must be admitted to the hospital where they are taken off of all medication "cold turkey." Processes such as these can be very painful and uncomfortable for the patient. Those trying to recover from such addictions could occupy hospital beds that could potentially be filled with people that may have an ailment more serious than an addiction caused by a doctor. As an owner of a hospital, this is simply common sense from a moral standpoint. Assuming that an owner of a hospital's primary concern would be to help the general public, keeping space for those with more concerning ailments should be a top priority. Investigating pain management clinics and taking the necessary actions to either shut the clinic down, or morph the clinic into a viable option for patients to learn techniques outside of medication to deal with their pain[, is crucial].

Those affected by chronic pain are not limited to elder adults with numerous other health problems and concerns. In fact, a rise in chronic pain has been seen among younger people (Leger). Obviously chronic pain can have a significant impact on the lives and well-being of both demographics, but it is arguable that helping with young people affected by chronic pain should be one of the top priorities. Young people, especially those attending college, are spending their time collecting vital skills in order to be successful in their chosen career path. Usually when one is affected by addiction of a substance, they are unable to function in their daily life. Even those simply taking medication such as oxycodone are unable to operate machinery. This would include driving a car. Pain management clinics that do not teach alternate methods, especially to young people, are not allowing them to "live their life by the fullest." People that have [become] addicted to powerful medication are deprived from their everyday life and are not able to function in the real world. How would a college-bound teenager be able to learn the life skills that they need to successfully work and raise a family in today's society if they are unable to function while attending college or even high school? One could argue that special accommodations can be made, such as a teen attending college close to home. How can teenagers expect to become self-sufficient while they have to be watched over by their family as if they were a small child? As Tracy Smith labeled clinics in her article title, pill mills and pain management clinics are a "scourge" (Smith). Such clinics only spread the disease of addiction to those among all demographics, and suck the life out of valuable people in society. It is strongly recommended that across the nation, all pain management clinics should be investigated to ensure that they are not spreading such a plague to desperate patients. If one were to be discovered, not only the doctors that "treat" the patients, but the owners—from small business to corporation-size hospitals—would be held responsible as well.

Works Cited

Alvarez, Lizette. "Florida Shutting Pill Clinics." *The New York Times*. *The New York Times*, 31 Aug 2011. Web. 28 Mar 2012.

CBS. "Fighting the Scourge of 'Pill Mills'" CBSNews. CBS interactive, 16 Oct 2011. Web. 28 Mar 2012. <http://www.cbsnews.com/2100-3445_162-20121033.html>.

Leinw, Donna. "States Target Prescriptions by 'Pill Mills.'" *USA Today*. Gannett, 25 Oct 2011. Web. 28 Mar 2012. <http://www.usatoday.com/news/nationistory/2011-10-13/pill-rnill-drugtrafiickinW50896242/1>.

WcbMD. "Pain Management Clinic—Topic Overview." WebAID. WebMD, 10 June 2009, Web. 28 Mar 2012. <http://www.webrrid.com/pain-rnanagementfte/pain-management-clinic-topic-overview>.

Pain Presenting to the Emergency Room

Pain is inevitable. Suffering is optional

—Author unknown

by Brian K. Tomlinson, MMS PA-C

It is commonly known in the medical community that the complaint of pain is the most common reason that patients seek care in emergency department. Since 1987 I have worked as a physician assistant in urgent care and emergency medicine. I learned early on in my career that pain complaints are what emergency health care providers address almost every minute of their shift. Health care providers (physicians, physician assistants, and nurses) constantly monitor patient complaints, stories, facial grimaces, quirks, emotions, responses, and concerned family members.

As I began to write this chapter, I picked up the Sunday paper. The front page story was about how overdoses from prescription drugs are soaring.

In contrast, my literature research finds articles discussing how pain is not adequately treated by Emergency Departments.(ED). "Oligoanalgesia."

Hence, this defines the daily dilemma in the emergency department. Do we over treat or are we undertreating pain in our patients? Emergency departments across this country are faced with the task of seeing and evaluating more and more patients. It is no secret that EDs are increasingly overcrowded. The health care system has evolved to the point where the ED has become the doctor's office for many people. Right or wrong, this is the reality. It has become the dumping ground for many family doctors. Medicaid-pending patients and noninsured patients have no other choice other than to go to the ED. For whatever reason the patient presents to the ED, it tends to be for nonemergent complaints. More than sixty percent of ED patients have pain as their main symptom or a major part of their symptoms.[1] And many of these are chronic pain complaints. This poses the challenge for the health care provider in the ED.

When it comes to the subject of oligoanalgesia, it is hard to believe that many emergency medicine health care providers fail to acknowledge pain. Rather, our time is consumed with addressing pain complaints in our patients. There are regulatory standards that hospitals have to recognize. The Joint Commission on Accreditation of Healthcare Organizations (JCAHO) has standards in pain assessment and management.[2] These guidelines guarantee patients the right to effective pain management. Hospitals seeking accreditation see to it that these requirements are complied with. There are regulatory statutes on treating pain from the American College of Emergency Physicians (ACEP) as well. Given today's standards in medicine, it is difficult to imagine a patient's pain needs not properly addressed when they present to the ED.

To provide sufficient pain control, it is necessary to understand how to assess pain. A campaign promoting pain as the fifth vital sign began in the 90s. It is a tool to help the provider assess patient's pain. Having this understanding can facilitate efforts to treat the patient's pain. However, pain is subjective. Patients perceive pain differently. What causes agonizing pain to one person may only be moderate pain to someone else.

The truth is, the vast majority of ED patients are not "drug seekers," but seekers of pain relief. Health care providers look for the cause of the patient's pain, and the patient looks for the pain relief. According to

Dr. Kevin Stein, when a patient in pain enters the ED, he or she has two main concerns (not necessarily in this order):[1]

1. How quickly can I get relief from my pain?
2. What is causing this pain?

The major focus of health care professionals is:

1. What is the diagnosis?
2. What is the treatment for the underlying disease process?

It is easier to find men who will volunteer to die, than to find those who are willing to endure pain with patience.

—Julius Caesar

* * *

The frustration for the health care providers in the ED is when there is significant abuse of the emergency services for opioid (narcotic) gain. Drug-dependent patients do whatever it takes in order to feed their addiction. The problem is rampant. Increasingly, providers find themselves investigating patients' frequent ED visits. Looking up patients on PDMPs (prescription drug monitoring programs) can be time consuming. PDMPs are being introduced in many states. PDMPs summarize the controlled substances a patient has been prescribed, the practitioner who prescribed them, and the dispensing pharmacy where the patient obtained them. It is a warehouse of patient information for health care professionals, as well as it provides an important investigative tool for law enforcement.[3]

* * *

God heals and the doctor takes the fee.

Benjamin Franklin

Having worked in the ED for many years, I could share multiple anecdotes that involve patients going to extremes in order to get their fix. I have gotten to know some of these patients very well over the years. And some of them I know and see more of than some of my own family members.

It can be exhausting working in an environment where we often deal with the drug-seeking master manipulator. Determined patients will manipulate and argue until they get what they want. In dealing with these patients, the words often uttered out of frustration by the provider are, "I don't care, [do] whatever it takes to get them out of here." It is a sad fact. I call this "feeding the bears." And we all know what happens when you feed bears. They keep coming back.

I worked for a short time at a small suburban hospital. This hospital likens itself to a luxury hotel. I was astonished to see that there was such an increased concentration of drug-seeking behavior presenting to this small ED. There were shifts when almost every patient I saw was prescribed an opioid. During one very frustrating shift, I posed a question openly to the nurses standing in the nurses' station, "Is this all you do here, hand out mass quantities of pain medications?" It was silent for a second, and then almost in unison several of them said, YES! They were all frustrated. It was explained to me that this physician-owned hospital adopts "the patient is always right" philosophy. Patient complaints can trump the provider who attempts to exercise good, sound medical judgment. I'm aware of a physician that received a negative patient evaluation because he failed to fulfill the patient's desire to receive another milligram of a powerful narcotic called Dilaudid before he was discharged.

Feeding the bears keeps them coming back. But then the bears gradually become bold enough to tell the provider how to practice medicine. It leads one to wonder if the desire to produce high patient satisfaction scores contributes to this problem.

Water, air, and cleanness are the chief

articles in my pharmacy.

—Napoleon Bonaparte

* * *

I often tell my patients that if they find that they need more and more of the same thing, then perhaps it is not the solution to their problem. (I am referring to opioid pain medications.) Often patients don't look at other options in pain management. They seek out only the pills to ease their pain. They may escape it for awhile, but the problem never goes quite goes away. The attention is on this one aspect of their care. Their focus is usually aimed at a quick fix. They fail to be aware of many of the life-style choices in their life that need to change, changes that could purify their lives.

It's odd that you can get so anesthetized by your own pain or your own problemthat you don't quite fully share the hell of someone close to you.

—*Lady Bird Johnson*

* * *

I think Mrs. Johnson got this right. I was once witness to a woman (a known opioid and sedative abuser) when she was told that her granddaughter had nearly drowned and was hospitalized in critical condition. The grandmother's first response was, "Oh God! Why me?" There are patients who tend to focus on themselves. They dwell only on their problems. They lose sight of the world around them. The patient's mental and physical health would benefit greatly if they would become inclined to focus on the needs of others. Volunteering ones time and caring for others can be a powerful pain reliever. Giving of oneself to others can promote the release of pain-relieving endorphins.

I have found the paradox, that if you love until it hurts, there can be no more

hurt, only more love.

—*Mother Teresa*

* * *

Patients need to accept the fact that life is not painless. And they need to accept the reality that their body changes with age. No one is entitled to a painless existence during this walk on earth.

I firmly believe that everyone has a story. And when they present to the ED, they need to tell their story. And they need to be heard. As health care providers, we become professional listeners. It's what we do. We listen to people's problems day in and day out. I never discount or minimize any patient who presents to the ED with pain. I tell the students I mentor,

"Always give the patient the benefit of the doubt and listen to their story completely, it will serve you well."

Rarely do you meet a patient who possesses the tools they need in order to cope with their pain. They need direction. We as health care providers need to lead them in the right direction.

On a personal note; when I am inflicted with pain, I hold onto my deep, childlike faith and pray often. I offer up my pain to the lost souls. I find much truth in these last two quotes:

If you suffer, thank God! It is a sure sign that you are alive

—*Elbert Hubbard*

* * *

Pain is never permanent.
—Teresa of Avila

* Emergency Department Protocols (complete article) by Kenny Stein, MD. Kenny Stein, MD, board certified in internal medicine, is an assistant professor for St. Louis University, Division of Emergency Medicine. In addition, he is an attending physician at St. Anthony's Medical Center in St. Louis. His interest in pain management has led him to lecture nationally on acute and chronic pain and JCAHO Pain Management Standards.

* Essential Elements of Effective Pain Management, Joint Commission Resources. 2001.

THE PATIENT'S STORY: MY INTERPRETATION

The experience of my patient certainly approaches that of patient abuse, mental torture, malpractice, assault on one's being, perhaps even a horror story. Unfortunately, I have heard the scenario many times before from other patients, some even worse. I've witnessed this for years from the same pain centers. I remind people this does not go on in every pain center, perhaps fifty percent of them, but honestly, that's being conservative. I'm afraid I have to lump them generally together because the good ones are not doing anything about the bad ones. Even though they have the most knowledge to do it, they are not participating in fixing this very serious problem. I'm on my own!

Some of the other stories I've heard are well documented in my previous book, *The Fraud of Chronic Pain*. That tells it frankly enough, doesn't it? Some of the patients are afraid to write their story because they would lose the source of their prescription. People can see their point; they are completely mentally dependent on it. It is very difficult for addicts to help themselves; probably only ten to twenty percent are ever cured of the problem. People can see why prevention is so important. A number of Medicaid taxi drivers hear the conversations in the backseat of their taxis. People may not realize it, but economically deprived or disabled patients are provided a taxi service free from their home to the provider and back—another way the government is helping many of the addicts to become addicted further. They're going to the pain center, they don't cure addiction, and they cause it and promote it. As the patient mentioned in the story, many of the people sitting in the waiting room are out there to get the narcotic and then sell it on the street. They get the prescription legally; they are "the legal addict" and narcotic salesman.

Medicaid drivers are not that anxious to tell the story because they might lose their job. Although I have been working on it, the written story has not come through.

Let's follow the story a bit closer in case you didn't understand some of the terminology or you don't know exactly what these medications do. Kadian, Opana, Norco, methadone, Fentanyl, Percocet, morphine, and OxyContin are all highly addictive opiate medications.

I'll explain what pain actually is, as well as what the habituation and addictive process is, in the following chapters. It's important to one's life because narcotics are handed out by hospital ERs, pain centers, provider's offices, and pain centers almost like they're candy, except they're expensive. There is great difference of opinion regarding how fast the addictive process is. Then again, everyone agrees one can become addicted in one week, and you may be one of them. For some people it may take even longer. A good eighty percent of people will never get off the medication, ruining their lives in the meantime; some will die in the addictive process.

When did my patient's habituating and addictive process begin?

The first mistake was made by the physician who gave her Vicodin after an injury at work that was not clear. There were no external signs of injury; he never even took an x-ray to see if there were internal causes. She said she had pain and that was it. I would like to make it perfectly clear where the big mistake was: narcotics should not be given to a person when they don't fully know where the pain is located. No clear cause, no narcs. It was a big mistake!

However, people might say, "But she went to work!" We can all work no matter what when we have enough of the feel-good hormone dopamine on board. That's perfectly understandable, but we are not considering the potential consequences. At least the patient should have had an endpoint, let's say a month.

She became hyperactive on the Vicodin, typical of narcotics and alcohol, which stimulate the glutamate system deep in the nervous system. Then she quit her job. Why? It was the effect of narcotics on her nervous system. She went to an orthopedic surgeon, who ordered physical therapy—fine. Then he made a mistake: he sent her to the pain center when he didn't even know why she had the pain, and he should have been the expert on causes of pain, especially with a work-related injury! He didn't know why she hurt and he sent her for pain treatments. Not very smart. So what starts the addictive process? The orthopedic doctor knows the pain doctor will stick needles in her to make their money, but he's rid of her: talking doesn't pay much. Then the pain doctor says pain pills will give people a better quality of life! There is an ignorant statement. Every physician knows narcotics are addictive and yet they hand them out like candy. They will not lead to a better quality of life!

The next doctor put her on Fentanyl—twenty times stronger than morphine and very addictive, especially when taken for centralized, cerebral, chronic pain. It is meant for acute or chronic pain when we know the reason. Acute pain tells people what the problem is. Then they did procedures on her: spinal blocks—needles in her back, really deep, potentially dangerous, started to burn some of her nerves in the spinal column. When people don't know what they are treating, what good is that? We still don't know what is wrong. No wonder the pain gets worse! Besides the fact that they gave her addictive drugs, they are also burning her nerves and causing real nerve damage. There was no real nerve injury until now, or so it seems; no one knows for sure. X-rays are negative. Maybe it's nothing. They turn around and give her morphine. Morphine, when given for an unclear cause, is very addictive—again, a major error!

Now the family doctor gets involved with the case too. He starts injecting her all over the body; he's known for that. I've never known a family doctor who does it to that extent. She's screaming there, like it's a form of torture. And we still don't know why she hurts! Now he sends her to another doctor as a reward. She calls him "the god." I know the man myself; I can see the point. He orders another MRI but nothing is found. So why treat? How about for money? He does spinal injections and again burns her nerves, which makes things worse; he makes a lot of money, thousands. The patient is no better and the addictive process is only promoted to make sure she comes back for a refill. What would one call this? Is it abuse, crime, fraud, malpractice, or good medical care? You decide.

Then he starts her on OxyContin—we all know where that goes—and it promotes a craving and produces a tremendous high. We all could use some of that. She's given a choice of three drugs: OxyContin, methadone, or morphine. Pathetic and abusive. These are all highly addictive narcotics, some more than others, and methadone builds up a half-life—in other words, it stays in one's blood and accumulates. This makes for a very dangerous situation; some people just die in their sleep because of it. I know specific cases where this happened.

Can you imagine giving a habituated-addicted person a choice of narcotics? That's criminal. This doctor's office is an opium den. My patients call pain centers "cash cows that addict people," and I've heard that more than once. Actually, the medical professionals have known about their abusive tactics for years and nothing has been done. Awareness of fraud and not reporting it may even be against the law; I am not sure about that.

This doctor did every possible procedure to her, although they x-rays were negative. Does that make sense to anyone? Actually, with the treatment of the pain, the pain gets worse. Does that tell you something? Some would even blame the patient, but that's ridiculous. She's addicted, she really has centralized brain pain, but they're treating the spine because it "pays." This is workman's comp; many providers make money from that.

She was also on sleep medication because she became hyperactive from the narcotics. They continued to increase the OxyContin medication; she had a storage bag full of medications. Does that give anybody a clue?

They kicked her out of this clinic because she was using the medications too fast, typical of addicts. I'm also acquainted with this office. Multiple offices, lot of pain doctors. Of course, he wanted to perform a procedure right away; that's the key to unlock the door to the narcotics. He was adamant about the injections, and I wonder why? Money. She thought she was out of her mind at this point; they of course burned her nerves, more injections, more pain, but it was the "key" to get the narcs. No injections, no narcs. Lots of pain. She was prescribed Kadian, a highly addictive opioid. It was slowly increased over time because of sensitization to the brain cells. She continued building receptor sites on the cells; these receptors are constantly hungry. She was also prescribed and taking Vicodin and OxyContin for breakthrough pain—pain medicines between Kadian doses. What a nightmare, a horror story.

Off to another pain clinic; they'd made the money already so they kicked her out of this one, probably also because of not following the rules—let's face it, very few addicts follow the rules. They did not treat her main problem, drug addiction. This center even has a psychologist on staff now but does not appear to be doing much good. Did I say you can't cure drug addiction while addicting a person with increased doses?

Now she goes to another pain clinic in an orthopedic office. They do a discogram, injecting a disc with a needle and running a test. We neurosurgeons know that's a very unreliable test. They say it's positive and she gets an operation. Of all things, the surgeon does a lumbar fusion. No sign of instability, no dislocation, no fracture, and no evidence of a ruptured disc on the MRI. Let's face it: she was just assaulted by the surgeon.

As expected, it didn't do any good, it made her even worse. Wonder why? If a person actually has a large rupture in a disk, then well-demonstrated or diagnostic studies, clear-cut neurological findings, and results from surgery are just great. But if surgeons operate on normal people and addicted people, they're going to make things worse, as in this case. An operation was not what she needed. She needed psychiatric counseling.

She was placed on Opana again, a highly addictive drug. Again, the medication was increased as far as she could take it. She felt the end was coming. She started staying in bed all day. Her son, who was stealing her drugs, taught her how to "snort" the drug. The drug is more rapidly absorbed if people put it up the nose, because the blood vessels are on the surface. It works a lot faster. She's a "legal addict" and now she's a "street addict" too, all created by the physician prescription. No relatives or family, no work, in bed all day, no church, and she felt like she was in the process of dying. She called her mother in Florida. Her mother agreed to pay $10,000 to put her in a drug treatment center run by a wonderful group of previously addicted females. They clearly helped her. She then started counseling at one of the local hospitals which is known to run a good drug rehab center. Nevertheless, unbelievably, the counselor sent her back to a pain center in her facility. A major mistake. The situation was saved though by the patient herself, because she was educated in the rehab hospital in

Florida never to touch a narcotic again. She refused to take the narcotic prescription offered to her by that pain center in the hospital, when that doctor clearly knew she had been at a rehab center in Florida. To me, it clearly would be malpractice to offer a narcotic to an addicted rehabilitative patient when people don't even know why they hurt. The Supreme Court ruled in 1919 that giving a narcotic to an addicted person is a crime! A major mistake. Fortunately, the patient refused. She described the waiting room of that pain doctor. Again, nothing but an opium den. People selling drugs, a narcotic mill. She had to run out of that pain clinic. Her description is like that of Dante's hell. It was a mill.

What is a person to do about this? Just walk away? Write a book, contact the medical society, contact the county government, contact the mayor, contact the state government, the state medical society, or contact the Feds? I've done that!

The Fraud of Pain

The prescription of narcotics for chronic pain by providers and especially pain clinics has reached epidemic proportions. This is occurring all over the country, in some states more than others. Just recently in a southern Ohio county, clinics were closed by the government. Owners are facing prosecution in the courts. These were nothing but procedure and narcotic mills. Weekly and almost daily, we read about pain clinic closures from all over the country, especially Florida. Ohio and Florida have passed laws regulating the number of pain centers. I say hallelujah to that. Also, laws are being passed in the state of Washington.

What's the motivation? The customers are looking for "dopamine" to feel good. Many are economically deprived. The owners of these clinics, of course, are largely doing it for the money, and many earn millions. Some providers have multiple offices in surrounding counties. Some even own MRI scanners when in reality there are many in the neighborhood. I wonder what their indications are. Of course, not all of the pain centers are the same. Some do very little of this, although I know of only two or three. Form your own opinion after reading my patient's story. What a business! We would all like to sell something that the buyer would become addicted to—return business is guaranteed! If people sold dopamine, serotonin, and endorphins and Medicare/Medicaid would even pay for it, what a business that would be. A majority of these patients in the pain centers are on Medicaid, and guess what? They don't even have a deductible. They don't even have to pay for their own gas to get there. The government pays for the taxi, picks people up and takes people home. Some of these taxi drivers listen to the conversations, and guess what? The customers talk about where to sell the medication. I have heard that story from many drivers. OxyContin is sold on the street for $40 to $80 a pill. One hundred pills would make people about $8000...wow! The scandal is that they are creating addicts, ruining lives. People who do the best have about a twenty percent chance of ever getting off all of the medications. The majority are actually taking multiple medicines, including tranquilizers and seizure medications, because narcotics sensitize the brain, causing seizures. Tranquilizers and sleeping medications become necessary in many of these patients. Many have multiple injuries because of falls that occur when they are doped up with medicine. Many are involved in accidents, and many also smoke and drink alcohol to calm their nerves.

A three-star army general, General Fridavich, was quoted in *USA Today* saying that thirty percent of his troops who had seen an army physician in Tampa were addicted to narcotic medication. Just think of the illness and cost to the army and VA system over the years—astronomical! I called him and met with him in Naples about a year ago. I offered to help the army with this project, but they declined. I think they realized that a lot of veteran benefits are based on disability. I'm guessing that's the reason, but people can see the motivation. I've called the general a number of times since. I think in his heart he wanted to act, but I think the surgeon general of the army is stopping him. That's speculation on my part. I offered to become an employee of the army to stop this horrible addiction rate, to design the program for the soldiers. I must say, though, that the general did give me a medal for my work.

I see these people from the pain center every day in my practice and they become habitually addicted to drugs. Of course, many also have had multiple unsuccessful procedures done to their back and many have previous back surgeries that were based on wrongly interpreted x-rays. Certainly not all of them, but many. These people now have another diagnosis called chronic pain. The brain has been changed, and then the receptors of the brain are different.

Chronic Pain: "I Hurt"

The definition of pain and how the patient and providers interpret it, I think, is confusing and mistaken. Acute pain causes only about ten percent of pain problems. It points out where the problem is. If people fix it, the pain goes away. Acute pain has an endpoint: fix the problem and it's over. Chronic pain is a horse of another color. It's pain that lasts more than six months, and generally the cause of the pain is unknown. Chronic pain is divided into neuropathic pain, nociceptive neuropathic pain, and metabilic pain (centralized brain pain). The latter two are about ten percent each. That leaves us with seventy percent of the chronic pain with no name. Idiopathic pain…who wants to be an idiot, pathetic? The last three pain books I read don't even have a name for the seventy percent of pain that is left over. They think the majority is neuropathic pain, pain based on nerve damage, but they are dead wrong. The majority of chronic pain is due to anxiety, anger, depression, hopelessness, and fear. The Buddhist would call this "arrow two" pain, arrow one being acute pain and arrow two referring to the emotion, the meaning, and the perception of the pain. In other words, we are speaking about pain that has been decorated by the human mind, and what do the pain centers do? They stick needles in patients and habitually addict them to drugs. An industry that makes a lot of money has been created with national associations to back them. The Joint Commission of Hospital Associations even backed them up by establishing the fifth vital sign. The fifth vital sign can be the beginning of narcotic habituation and addiction. In the emergency room, what is the first question they ask you? "What's the level of your pain on a scale from 0 to 10"? Not, "What is the cause of your pain, what's going on in your life?" The patient should be handed a yellow pad and a pencil to write their story and avoid unnecessary treatment. Health care providers would be much more likely to make a correct diagnosis. The treatment of chronic pain, in my opinion, is frankly abusive, with many unnecessary injections and millions of unnecessary prescriptions. We are creating a "pain society"; we are a pain nation. That is where the Joint Commission of Hospital Associations with that fifth vital sign, along with the pain centers, has carried us. The psychiatrist in the hospital is even more upset than I am because they treat the final product. In about ten chronic pain consultations today, people will become addicted through the narcotic prescription in the quest for a quick fix. What if Florida, Ohio, and Washington established new state laws outlawing the further development of pain centers? Could this be a sign of the future? Makes you wonder. Florida has the most generous workman's comp laws in the nation. They pay for minor disabilities and of course the major ones, where frankly the payments are needed for a lifetime. Certainly for the latter it's very helpful, but for the addicted patient it is a life of misery, even though they get a workman's comp check for the rest of their life. Many lead useless lives. I suspect the pain center celebrated when that person first came in for help, because a lot of disabilities are based on pain. Pain centers made addicts out of these injured people and have guaranteed a lifetime customer. What a business.

Are We Supposed to Be Healers?

We need an endpoint for the narcotic prescription. Acute pain has value: people fix it and it should be over. Chronic pain does not do much for us: "I hurt but I don't know why." Some providers want to call chronic pain a disease. It is not. It's a sensation, a symptom, an emotion or perception. It's only a disease if we hand out narcotics to the patient and don't use some other method to treat them. In pharmacological research, it has been shown that narcotics work only thirty percent of the time in thirty percent of the people. That is a well-known fact. So I say to people, why do they prescribe narcotics for long-term pain when those drugs can cause a lot of damage? I like to call the seventy percent of pain whose cause is unclear "metabolic pain (centralized brain pain)," This is a term I just made up to give it a reasonable name. Certainly it's better than "idiopathic pain." We know why people hurt—it's anxiety, fear, depression, hopelessness, and anger. We can't just ask for the level of one's pain because it creates lifetime addiction, unless people have acute pain or cancer. At least we have a name for "metabolic pain" for the patient with centralized brain pain rather than something made up based on x-ray readings, like a degenerative disease or bulging disc, when actually it's nothing to do with the problem. We're doing a "nocebo" to the patient, known as "negative speak," the opposite of the placebo. We make up things on diagnostic tests and relate them to the pain when actually it has nothing to do with it. I see that every day and that is for what people have to watch out. That's why people need other opinions. This is especially so in the pain business. Remember, seventy percent of pain problems, the "bumps and bruises of life," are real but based on anger, fear, hopelessness, anxiety, and depression. It's a perception. Not decorating the pain and becoming mindful by removing the baggage can help a great deal. The shot in one's back and narcotics as a reward are not going to do it. Don't accept narcotics for metabolic chronic pain. As consumers, people need to be very careful about this. Addiction to drugs is rampant. Most medical providers, unfortunately, have no understanding of how to treat chronic pain. I do know that some of the practices are totally dependent on writing narcotic prescriptions or just want the patient out of the office. In a neighboring county, three physician practices do nothing but write out opiate prescriptions for pain. A physician who covers the practices when they're on vacation or on the weekends has told me this. Patient satisfaction is what they're looking for in the emergency room. What's the level of one's pain on a scale of 0 to 10? That's a patient's key to the world of narcotics; they're now a legal addict. I realize that when people are in pain, even if it's metabilic pain (centralized brain pain), the pain is real and it is difficult to motivate people to seek a second opinion. However, think of the future. Drug addiction is not the way to go; one's life will be ruined. Read my book *The Fraud of Chronic Pain* and you will have the knowledge to avoid this plague. The book could be a second opinion. Pain will not kill people, but narcotics do it regularly. The Buddhists speak of arrow one pain—acute pain, the pain itself. Arrow two pain is the decorating of that pain by anger, depression, fear, hopelessness, and anxiety. People are actually suppressing it with drugs, alcohol, and cigarettes. You need to be mindful of your pain and stop decorating it or you will drown in it. Mindfulness teaching, as described in my book, treated with holistic healing methods, is the answer. People must participate in their own healing to get the job done. A "quick fix" with narcotics, opiates, or tranquilizers only makes it permanent.

The Hidden Epidemic

Many cultures don't even allow narcotics to be routinely used for pain problems. Pain has been interpreted differently across the cultures.

Abuse of pain medication through physicians' narcotic prescriptions is occurring throughout the country, some places more than others. A war is going on. There were fifteen thousand deaths from physicians' narcotic prescriptions in 2011. Many people die silently in the night: thirteen hundred in Ohio last year, and seventy in our surrounding counties three years in a row. I personally know of friends who have lost children through narcotic additictions, which started through valid prescriptions. We are developing a nation of pain.

We need national leadership to attack this problem, but I don't expect it to happen because there's too much money involved. I don't think the national pain societies will get it done because of financial motivation. I would think the legitimate and holistic pain centers should form a separate organization and vigorously attack the problem because they may be swept up in the legislation from the state or federal government. For example, in an Ohio county, all the pain clinics were closed. That would not be right either, but how could a civil agency tell the difference between the centers? It takes an experienced medical person to do that. Turning all the pain problems over to the pain centers would be a major error.

Unnecessary surgery is part of the problem. When the patient doesn't get better, he is sent to a pain doctor. Unfortunately this occurs frequently in the family doctor's office because the doctor doesn't have the time to deal with a patient's chronic pain, and the patient is sent to a pain center when there is no clear cause of pain. Frankly, I get the point, but many times this adds to the addictive process. They would be better off by personally dealing with the patient, but many times it is impossible to talk an addicted patient into holistic healing. Prevention really is the key, and that's why I do what I do. Did anyone notice that at the end of her story, my patient had a totally unnecessary spinal fusion? No dislocation, no fracture, no instability, essentially nothing on her x-rays.

Pain today is different than it was in the time of our ancestors. We used to have the baby and go back to work. A friend of mine was visiting the delivery room area in a hospital in Kenya; it was the quietest room in the hospital. What can you say? It's all about perception. Perception, expectation, emotions, and fear mean everything.

The societal forces promoted this change in perception and are as powerful as gravity.

The difference between acute and chronic pain in modern and ancient times is huge. When Dr. David B. Morris first walked into a pain clinic and witnessing the doctors in white coats, he thought he was witnessing a group of imposters. It gave him the authenticity, dominion over people. As my wife said to me one day, "You think you're God." The patient may mistakenly interpret a doctor's position that way, but I know what I am.

The most insidious factor is that we don't recognize that this is an epidemic. It's a very quiet one that addicts and kills people. Chronic pain escapes notice most of the time. We have medicalized pain; we spend billions on it yearly. It started in 1890 or so with aspirin and then the use of ether around 1846. This was a great discovery for acute pain. But it's chronic pain, pain lasting longer than six months, that is ninety percent of the problem.

After the discovery of ether, pain didn't die. The situation only became worse.

The pain clinics are filled with people whose lives have changed. Just reading descriptions from a patient sitting in the waiting room of a pain clinic is very distressing to me. It should be to everyone, but especially for those in the medical community. The room is full of habituated, addicted, depressed, largely economically deprived people. When I walked by a pain clinic recently, I looked past the glass wall and it was like a concentration camp. Remember, I lived in Germany during the war. Most people in the clinic were poorly dressed; the ones walking by me or on the elevator with me to the clinic had the odor of smoke and stared straight ahead. My patients have described images like this to me many times and I personally have witnessed it. When people watch these patients move, they don't see them limping; they don't appear to be physically disabled. It's the centralized pain in their mind that is destroying them, largely promoted by the procedures and prescriptions, by hopelessness, stress, anxiety, depression, and the bumps and bruises of their lives.

Yesterday while making rounds when I was on call for neurosurgery, I met the new head of the trauma section at a new hospital. I liked him immediately. We spoke about how pain is treated in Europe and in Egypt. He had worked in all those areas. In Egypt, no narcotics were prescribed when people left the hospital unless they had cancer. Guess how many people there have become addicted through their physician's prescription? Essentially zero. He tells me that in Germany it was the same. None of this issue in the hospital, "What is the level of your pain, 0 to 10?" These other doctors actually asked, "Where do you hurt?" or "Why do you hurt inside?" to discover the real cause.

Chronic pain is especially treacherous because it works mainly in secret. I saw a patient on Friday who had a pain problem. He had a minor back injury years ago. No ruptured disks, no broken back. He was started on narcotics, and then they placed a pain pump, delivering morphine via catheter right into the spinal fluid of the spinal cord so that it is rapidly absorbed into the nervous system. He was now completely dependent on it and was treated with a second narcotic that did not give the usual high and craving. Then again, it was just another narcotic which he will have to stay on, probably for ever. He felt good enough to work. That's completely ridiculous. I'm certain the pain doctor thought he had a great result, and I know the patient thought he had a great result. Personally, I think it's almost criminal. We have created a disease in him called chronic pain. He should have been treated conservatively with exercise and stress reduction. He is habituated and probably addicted to narcotics. We all would like to have some more dopamine every day, but how about exercise, laughter, and some music in our lives?

There was nothing on this patient's x-rays that warranted that sort of treatment. He just said, "I hurt, my level of pain is an eight," and narcotics were started. A disgusting way to treat people, especially by a healer.

Many of the patients have had back surgery—that's fifty percent of the pain people's business. Many have had two to three operations. Many of those went to the surgeon with their MRI scan showing the process of aging and somebody made a disease out of it. The radiologist may have created a two- to five-page report of every single little thing on the x-ray which actually had little to do with the patient's complaint. A much better question than "Where do you hurt?" might have been "What's going on in your life?" The over-reading of MRI scans by radiologists and surgeons is common. I'm ashamed to admit it, but it is reality.

The public, the medical community, and yes, even the insurance companies are not aware that many CT and MRI scans are not reliable. They are just great for some things like tumors. But the rest of time they can be very confusing. Everybody thinks a bulging disc means something. It means very little, but it is used as the excuse (nocebo) to inject and operate on somebody every single day. The public is not aware. Insurance companies are not aware. Surgeons and pain centers are aware, but need an excuse to do something because that's where the money is!

I had something happen to me recently. Our corporate manager handed me a letter of complaint from a patient who had sent my consultation fee back to the insurance company. The insurance company thought I should've operated on the patient. The things they underlined on the x-ray report were in reality just the normal changes one would see in a person of that age and weight. I told the patient she did not need an injection or surgery. I even demonstrated to her how to exercise and to lose some weight and gave her a free book to read on stress. Her child was also obese. I spent over thirty minutes with them. I think she was looking for a quick fix. One would think the insurance company would appreciate what I tried to do, but in essence they said I should've operated on her. My manager fell for it and sent the consult fee back, when in reality I had given her great advice. The insurance industry doesn't even understand or want to understand the overtreatment of pain by pain clinics and surgeons and the public who want a quick fix. A very sad situation. What is a reasonable man to do? I guess write books!

Chronic pain is the perception of the patient. It's different in every culture, race, and society. The patient sitting quietly in the waiting room, staring straight ahead, with no visible sign of pain, experiencing pain that is mainly centralized in the brain most of the time, is certainly real. But this pain is created largely by anxiety, fear, depression, and anger, and the narcotic prescription makes it permanent. It is extremely difficult to cure these people, although it can be done with a lot of work. The chronic pain problem is perpetuated by the narcotic prescription and decorated with emotions, fear, and anxiety, and many times it ruins a person's life. It's a war.

Neuropathic chronic pain is actually created by nerve damage. It accounts for only about ten percent of pain problems and serves no purpose. It does not warn people of anything that might save their lives, nor does it tell them where the problem is. It's invisible.

Since about twenty to thirty percent of the pain clinics are more reasonable and legitimate, I hate to lump them together. By the same token, they have not formed an association that is doing something about the horrible clinics that are addicting people, taking their money, and ruining their lives. Unfortunately, all of these clinics will get lumped together as a potential solution is sought. I think these clinics should have formed their own associations and tackled this problem so that others like myself don't have to do it. Certainly the government is starting to partially wake up and get involved with these clinics from a narcotic standpoint. But government is not looking at it from a procedure or pain standpoint. The solution should not be the responsibility of the government, it should be the holistic pain doctors organizing and starting a war on the scam artists. I'm afraid that is not going to happen, though; there's too much money in the whole process. Even the reasonable pain clinics are making the money from injections. They may think they're being conservative, but when I really look at them, they're not. They don't truly believe in the centralized theory of pain. They couldn't exist without procedures. But it's the fault of the insurance companies who won't pay for conservative measures. They won't even pay $200 for a member to join an exercise club. They would much rather pay $100,000 for an unnecessary back operation or spinal injection. I know a pain clinic where they do thirty to a hundred spinal blocks a day, at a cost of $1000 to $2000 each, and then they hand the patient an opiate prescription to be sure he comes back for a refill, after which they recommend another periodic spinal injection because the patient's not going to get better as long as he's addicted. Believe me, I see that every day.

We need a new "definition of pain." No narcotics for centralized or what I call "metabilic pain (centralized brain pain)." I don't think we'll see that happen. There's too much money in the current system. I recommend that seventy five percent of the pain clinics be closed by the government, and the rest must treat pain with a new definition. Insurance companies must pay for modalities like yoga, exercise, Zumba, massage, dance, art and music, weight-loss classes, and stress-reduction classes. There are billions of dollars involved in this industry, but won't hold my breath till reform has taken place.

The state governments of Florida, Ohio, and Washington are at work creating legislation that controls and closes down a lot of these clinics. On the other hand, how does one separate the good ones from the bad ones? I think all pain clinics need to be painted with a brush that might illuminate some of the good ones. I don't see how that is avoidable.

A member of the city council in Seattle wanted to put all pain treatment under the responsibility of all the pain clinics. That would have been a horrendous mistake. We could addict the whole country! We have just about done that already, but believe me, it could even get worse.

Most chronic pain is pain in the brain and difficult to prove with one hundred percent certainty. Pain patients are difficult to deal with because all they want is a refill. Trying to reason with them is an impossible situation, even in my conservative experience. So who is going to do it? Psychiatrists are tired of it. There are billions of dollars involved and the pain industry is not going to let go of that money without a fight. Certainly the government is not up to it, they have no experience with it. Let's face it, psychiatrists also hand out a lot medication—talking doesn't pay! The neural anatomy and neurochemistry are difficult to understand, so one can see the problem.

One has to look at the big picture. No one dies from pain. There were probably fifteen thousand deaths from physician pain prescriptions last year. One easily can see the difference. What is easy to understand, though, is the rate of habituation and addiction when one speaks to psychiatrists. The psychiatrist at my hospital who sees these patients in routine consultations every day is even more adamant than I am about this problem. I asked him to step up to bat, but he refused.

Dr. David B. Morris says, "It's never as simple a matter of nerves and nerve transmitters, but pain needs to be interpreted in terms of the personality, cultural setting, and meaning." He also says that it certainly proves the past four or five generations that we have been living with an organ model of pain. Medicine is now the industrial complex. Pain has moved from the household into the marketplace. Today the most innovative work in contemporary pain treatment suggests that the old organic model needs a major overhaul. One researcher examined the records of ten thousand patients with back injuries from 1977 in the state of Washington. Patients with low back pain account for one third of all worker's compensation cases and received $64 million in compensation.

Pain entered the marketplace. Seventy five percent of the patients had no findings of real organic pathology. Examinations and x-rays were negative. If they want to, doctors can find changes on an MRI scan in every spine of every living thing except very young children. This is used as the excuse to do things to people, and the public is not aware of that. The ones looking for a quick fix will not be believe that the changes on the x-rays mean nothing. They don't say, "Wonderful, I don't even want an operation!" The majority are looking for a quick fix, many times for psychological problems in their lives, and the injectors and operators are glad to oblige them. In the old days we had dye injected into the spine, and that test was a lot more honest. If the myelogram was normal, no surgery was done. But remember what I said, that MRI shows changes in almost everyone, the majority of which are normal changes of aging and mean very little.

The moral modern thinking in the future hopefully will be that chronic pain is a perception, has meaning, and should be studied in the context of what's going on in your life. The social context of the pain must be considered. The body has multiple pain pathways. They become especially important in acute pain because they indicate what the problem is. However, that's only ten percent of the pain problems.

Pain pathways include the brain, the autonomic nervous system, and the sympathetic and the parasympathetic nervous system, which influence the emotional limbic system that governs our emotions in the brain. This makes pain an emotional event, even in acute pain. How we interpret pain differs from one person to another. Pain is an emotion, perception, cognition, and a social, cultural setting.

In the future we are likely to see large numbers of doctors and patients supplementing or replacing the old organic model with the new multidimensional model. But don't hold your breath till it happens. The multidimensional model should encompass the intersection of physiology, emotional cognition, and the social aspects of pain.

Pain is more than a medical issue and has social and political connotations. Medicine probably will never change the definition; the legislatures of counties, states, and the country probably will need to step up to bat. They should outlaw narcotics for chronic centralized brain pain or

Metabolic Pain. That would stop the opioid epidemic and put the addiction doctors out of business. They have not earned our trust. It's unfortunate, and the pain centers will get caught up in the process.

The future will draw two very different pictures of pain. Seventeenth-century philosopher René Descartes, in his famous *Treatise of Man*, describes the original theory on pain: people break a toe and the pain impulse goes up a rope to the brain and rings the bell. That is essentially the way we are treating pain today—with no connection to the emotional part of our brain.

The Closing of Narcotic Mills

Pain clinics have been closed by the state governments in multiple states. We've all been reading about Florida closing pain clinics for a few years now. It is especially bad in Tampa. The legislature is passing laws that regulate these clinics, though I would think that is very difficult to do. There has been a particularly big problem with a lot of pain clinics according to my friend, three-star general Fridovich, whom I spoke with in Naples, Florida. His story has been well written up a national newspaper. He even gave me a friendship medal. I highly appreciated that. I gave the army a lot of education about chronic pain with CDs, DVDs, and books. But I think he found the politics of the army to be too complex to change the system. Thirty percent of his troops who had seen a physician in the services were drug addicts. That was right in the news report. I think General Fridovich found that the army was not willing to change; I suspect there's too much work and money involved. If people took away the narcotics, the compensation payments would be lower. Most veterans would get them for the rest of their lives, so you can see the problem—too much money involved. I read an article in a Florida newspaper saying that pain mills have moved because of lax laws in the state. Florida is clamping down on this problem!

In January of this year, the last pain clinic was closed in Scioto, a town in southern Ohio. One doctor had written fourteen thousand prescriptions that year. Obviously, he's going to face charges.

There's now a government narcotic prescription tracing system called INSPECT that trained providers can access. Now doctors can also tell when a patient is shopping around at many pain clinics at the same time. I use this service regularly. But it's not just a matter of people doctor-shopping. Providers must understand the difference between the central and peripheral theory for pain. We need a new definition of pain. I'm afraid the pain societies will never provide it.

Certainly some pain centers are better than others, some are worse than others. How is the public to know when the doctors don't even know? I must say, even the better clinics generally don't promote holistic treatments of exercise, yoga, music, laughter, and stress reduction. Just look at their websites. Procedures dominate the system, unfortunately. I heard one of the pain doctors say on one of his regular TV programs, "We've done over one thousand spinal pain implants." I would not be proud of that, because now they have programmed pain patients. All these procedures need adjustments.

Sometimes sites become infected, other implants need to be removed, and some doctors inject narcotics into the nervous system and create habituation and addiction. The patient may even be able to go to work, though this would be very rare in the pain business, because most want disability and they are still habituated addicted to the medicine. They are slaves to the system, and spinal implants rarely solve the problem.

In 2007 in Ohio, drug overdoses originating in narcotic prescriptions surpassed car crashes as the leading cause of death. That is so in many states. A lot of the government crackdown occurred because of drug overdoses and deaths. A law in Ohio now requires the state board of pharmacy to license pain clinic as distributors of "dangerous drugs." Get the point? We're supposed to be healers, not habituating and addicting people.

Most countries don't have pain clinics or use the context for routine pain problems. Are we a peculiar people? I think not. We are seeking dopamine and serotonin to overcome the stresses of our lives. We are trying to escape this world. I just had my dopamine with a game of tennis and music on the radio on the way home.

Descartes wrote in1650, "The impulse traveling from the site of injury to the brain produces pain just as a pulley at the end of a cord and then the ringing of a bell in the brain." That's the mechanistic theory of pain today that is promoted by the pain clinics.

Descartes was the inventor of the organ models of pain as evolved in the mid-seventeenth century. It gives us a picture of pain in a vacuum. What's the social context? The emotion? The perception? The meaning? Descartes' model is a statue, not a living thing. Where's the civilization? Pain is not a medical event! The diagnosis conveniently lets us forget the social context of our pain. Pain is a perception with meaning and an emotion which should be the new model of chronic pain. Descartes stripped away the civilization and culture surrounding the person. It is easy to understand why is it difficult to cure pain when the patient lives in a world dominated by multiple forms of hardship and distress over which they have no control. But that gives us no excuse to make them worse by addicting them to narcotics, ruining their lives, and doing procedures to them to make money.

The social history of patients with pain problems reads like a brutal soap opera. That's what I see every day, and then the pain centers are brutalizing these people. Most are on multiple medications and the government is paying for a lot of this medicine and is promoting addiction. So the government is also at fault. The majority of these patients are on Medicaid and wouldn't be at the clinic if the government didn't pay the bill. I think the government has skin in the game. Many pain patients have been through divorce, abuse, loss of job, bankruptcy, and poverty, and so have some of their children because they abuse them. Many are plagued by obesity, depression, type II diabetes, and hopelessness. Many die young; they are the cause of many accidents. When I passed the pain clinic today I saw some people lying on the floor crying. I suspect all the people sitting there were sharing their pain. One patient told me when they were sitting in the pain crowd in the waiting room of the pain center, the doctor wouldn't see some of the people because they had not paid their bill.

Pain crosses all racial and social lines but is concentrated more in the working class because they have more stresses. Chronic pain is not a significant problem in non-Western cultures. They have closer societies and their expectations are different. Women who have a baby expect to have pain and don't even cry out. So expectations play also a part.

Let's revisit the future. It is considered unethical medical practice to let a patient continue in pain. I totally agree with that. But should we continue to addict them or kill them in the process? I think not! We clearly need a new a different approach for pain, a safer, more holistic one.

What's the Future?

"To allow a patient to bear unbearable pain is unethical and may turn into an unethical medical problem." I agree with this statement to a point. I must know why they have the pain. Just saying "I hurt" only works for short period of time with me.

Acute injury is a neuropathic injury (nerve damage) or cancer. Of course, proper treatment for acute pain is very important. I do not hesitate to give very strong medication when necessary. But I know what kind of problem the patient has, I know the cause. I do not give narcotics for chronic pain without clear diagnosis or what I call metabilic pain (centralized brain pain), pain based on anger, depression, hopelessness, anxiety, etc. Otherwise people become permanent customers of pain medications, which make the nerve receptors in the brain cells grow. This occurs when the dosage of narcotics is consistently increased, and as a result a lot of other medications may also be required, like tranquilizers and epilepsy medications.

People need to be masters of their pain and not the slaves. This can be accomplished through positive thinking. Sitting in the waiting room of a pain clinic allows you to get the picture. It is the picture of depression.

What does the future hold for the person with chronic pain? Today's pain clinic generally is not the answer, with an occasional exception. Ten seconds of conversation with the provider, an injection, and a narcotic script is the typical scenario for most who seek assistance at a pain clinic. Medical staff there might perform thirty to a hundred blocks a day, shuttling people through like they were in cattle cars, like in a concentration camp, as one patient told me.

The risk of dealing with quacks is high because of the money involved. Unfortunately surgery is not far behind. Read *Nocebo the Evil Twin* by Dr. Rudy Kachmann. Insurance companies, Medicaid, and Medicare help promote this fraud by paying it for it. Wake up! Many clinics are not run by properly trained personnel. Great pain clinics are rare. Look at their websites. There is little evidence of holistic treatment methods, because those methods don't pay. I own a Mind-Body Institute inside a hospital in Fort Wayne, Indiana. No prescriptions. Instead I promote CDs, DVDs, audio books, books, and all sorts of wellness modalities, including yoga classes, regular lectures—many of them free, stress reduction classes, and mindfulness.

Dr. Morris says the postmodern pain patient needs to take charge of his own destiny. But I tell people to sit in the waiting room of the pain clinic and observe for a while. You know it's not going to happen.

Providers, government agencies, and insurance companies must take charge to change the system. The fault lies in asking doctors to take charge of something that is beyond the physical explanation. It's the meaning for the patient, the perception, that they themselves must take charge of. Certainly education needs to be huge part of this, probably largely by people who have little personal involvement and get properly paid for talking to patients.

Pain Myths

First of all, many medical providers treat pain patients in the long run just with addictive medications and mind-altering drugs, tranquilizers, and anti-depressants. They don't distinguish the acute pain from the chronic pain, which is a major mistake. They don't give it a strong run with integrative medicine. As I will discuss in another chapter, there are many modalities available. Just treating pain problems with addictive drugs is like treating heart disease just with angioplasty. Chronic heart disease is a diet disease most of the time. Chronic pain problems are largely related to the neuropeptides, hormones, and the neural circuitry of the human mind.

Second, patients can underestimate the power, soul, and spirit of their own minds. They underestimate their own healing power and may not be interested in an holistic approach to pain. This is a major mistake. Holistic methods can help manage any pain problem and can reduce pain fifty to one hundred percent most of the time. That has completely been my experience; I've seen it work in cancer patients, with whom I would certainly be a lot more generous with narcotic medication.

Third, some patients have been tricked by providers into thinking that they must learn to live with their pain. I completely disagree. Changing medications or introducing new medication can help many pain problems, and I've never seen a pain problem that could not be helped through a holistic approach with a willing doctor and patient. America's preferred method of pain relief, though, both by patients and providers, continues to be painkillers. This is a major error.

Fourth, I never tell a patient that they are faking the pain, even if I suspect they are. I also never tell them that pain is just in their head or due to some psychological problem. The patient reacts to accusations like these by getting angry, or feels guilty on top of their suffering. There is no good test to measure pain. Most people, doctors included, assume that pain is always the result of damage to the body tissues. Unfortunately, that is completely untrue. People may have completely negative tests, but pain can be caused by neuropeptides, hormones, and neurotransmitters—the communicators of the human body—and the neural circuits of the body can be changed by chronic pain, especially when it's left untreated.

Fifth, patients often believe that their bodies are in danger because they have pain. The reality is that when pain is chronic, all bets are off. Ongoing pain sometimes causes tissue damage, but is not very common. The fear of damage and illness that naturally attends pain may alter the nervous system, causing people to hurt even more. Chronic pain carries little physical threat unless it causes a psychological breakdown, and I suspect an occasional patient commits suicide because of this. But that is much more likely to occur if they are on narcotics.

Last, many patients believe there's a magic bullet of pain relief, and that's why they keep on doctor shopping. "I have to keep trying new doctors until I find the one who will fix me once and for all." Looking for the quick fix is common. Chronic pain is usually the result of several things going awry—mechanical, chemical, and neurological—and it is also affected by the state of one's soul. There's really no one simple solution that can penetrate to all layers of the pain. Usually people need integrative medicine, the combination of conventional and alternative therapies. There is synergy among the treatments that adds up to something bigger, to one's very own chronic pain solution.

* * *

The Neurobiology of Stress

"Future shock [is] the shattering stress and disorientation that we induce in individuals by subjecting them to too much change in too short a time."

—Alvin Toffler

* * *

Less than a century ago, the word "stress" wasn't a part of the American lexicon. Engineers working on the Brooklyn Bridge in Lower Manhattan understood the technical term as "mechanical forces acting on physical structures." According to linguist, author, and pundit William Safire, *stress* the noun is a shortening of *distress*, rooted in the Latin distringere, "to hinder, molest." *Stress* the verb has another root as well: the Latin stringere, "to draw tight, press together," which is related to strain. Today stress has come to take its meaning from the verb *pressure*: "whether through direct force, tension exerted on a person or thing." Pressure, tension, and stress, which are synonymous in general use, lead to anxiety and strain. The vogue term was presaged by John Locke circa 1698: "Though the faculties of the mind are improved by exercise, yet they must not be put to a stress beyond their strength."

Stress is the inability to cope with *perceived* (real or imagined) threats to one's mental, physical, emotional, and spiritual well-being, which results in a series of physiological responses and adaptations. Internal stressors can also be physical (infections, inflammation) or psychological. External stressors include adverse physical conditions (such as pain or hot or cold temperatures) or stressful psychological environments. Medically speaking, stress is the nonspecific response of the body to any demand. The presence of stress causes physical, measurable changes, such as an increase in pulse, respiration, and heart rate. Virtually all systems—cardiovascular, pulmonary, digestive, endocrine, immune, and nervous—act to meet the perceived danger. Stress has replaced infectious agents of disease as the number one health evil facing Western culture.

In the 1920s, physiologist Walter Cannon first used the term "stress" to describe the body's response to unpleasant conditions, named the "fight or flight response." In his classic *The Wisdom of the Body*, Cannon explained that the body had automatic control over functions such as temperature control, digestion, and heart rate. A single nerve called the vagus, which exits at the back of the brain and continues down the body via the spinal cord and nerve branches, can send signals to the body's organs, including the pupils of the eyes, the salivary glands, the heart, the bronchi of the lungs, the stomach, the intestines, the bladder, the sex organs, and the adrenal glands. When Cannon stimulated the vagus nerve through electrodes implanted in the brain's hypothalamus just above the pituitary gland, he discovered that there were physiological changes in all of these organs consistent with the body's response to an emergency. Blood, for example, was rerouted from the internal organs of digestion to the muscles. An increase of adrenaline stimulated the heart and caused the liver to release extra sugar for instant energy.

Acute stress stimulates the sympathetic adrenal system and an outpouring of adrenaline, like hormones that prepare the body for "fight or flight." Pupils dilate, blood pressure and heart rate rise, and blood flow to the brain increases, resulting in improved vision and other cerebral functions. Glycogen stores in the liver rapidly break down into glucose to provide immediate energy. Blood shunts from the gut to the muscles of the arms and legs so that we can run faster. Blood also clots more rapidly to diminish loss from any hemorrhage. In short, a host of potentially lifesaving physiological and chemical events occur under the body's stress response.

Hans Selye, a charismatic and influential neuroendocrinologist, popularized the notion that stress (and the emotional or physical reaction to it) can make people sick. Building on Cannon's model of the "fight or flight" response to a generalized notion of stress, Selye proposed that over time, harsh environments (including the stress of modern living) can cause increasing levels of physical stress, eventually resulting in physical syndromes, exhaustion, and even death. In his landmark study published in 1950, "The Physiology and Pathology of Exposure to Stress," Selye theorized that poor adaptation to stress was the basis of most illnesses and disease. His theories permeated medical thinking and influenced medical research for twenty years, replacing psychoanalytically based psychosomatic theories.

About ten years later, physicist Elmer Green developed biofeedback techniques in which patients learned to control unconscious processes.

Under his care, patients watched monitoring devices that tracked things like heart rate or blood pressure. By observing how their different actions affect data readouts, patients could start to voluntarily regulate certain body functions such as blood pressure. Green's experience led him to state,

"Every change in the physiological state is accompanied by an appropriate change in the mental emotional state, conscious or unconscious, and conversely, every change in the emotional state, conscious or unconscious, is accompanied by an appropriate change in the physiological state."

Herbert Benson found that under most circumstances, once the acute threat has passed, the response becomes inactivated and levels of stress hormones return to normal, a condition called the *relaxation response*. The problem is that contemporary life poses ongoing stressful situations that are not short-lived, and the urge to act (to fight or to flee) must be suppressed or the fight-or-flight response becomes perpetual. The physiology of stress and the fight-or-flight response has been studied and publicized more than any other neurochemical process. The body's stress response activates the brain's hypothalamus and pituitary glands, which regulate hormones, particularly the stress hormone cortisol that regulates immune functioning, blood pressure, insulin, and proper glucose metabolism. While small increases in cortisol improve performance, long-term (chronic) exposure to stress hormones can cause atrophy of the brain's hippocampus, leading to memory impairment. To make matters worse, we pour adrenaline into our bodies with cans of popular energy drinks; double-shot, three-pump grande cafe lattes; or exposure to popular movies and television shows— all of which cause our body and mind to endure even more stress. High cortisol levels also increase food intake and contribute to central body fat, a condition my colleagues in cardiology refer to as "toxic fat." Abdominal fat, insulin resistance or glucose intolerance, high blood pressure, inflammation and bad cholesterol are known to increase the progression of heart disease.

Prolonged stress also can be hazardous to brain function, hormone production, immune responses, and other processes. Stress-related disorders and diseases brought on or worsened by psychological stress commonly involve the autonomic nervous system, which controls the body's internal organs, including the heart, lungs, and brain.

Chronically stressed individuals have increased levels of the stress hormone cortisol, which slows the delivery of immune cells and molecules to injury sites. In turn, this slows the start of the healing process. In 2004, a twenty-year-long study proved that the longer the duration of a stressor, the greater the disruption

of pro-inflammatory cytokines, which in turn may increase susceptibility to viruses that cause the common cold. The study also showed that social relationships may influence wellness and recovery from disease. Social isolation such as loneliness raised blood pressure. Alzheimer's caregivers were more likely to have severe colds. Bereavement and unemployment lowered lymphocyte counts for up to two months after the initial stressor. Couples going through a divorce have depressed T and NK cells, immune cells that strengthen resistance to infection. And research on wound healing suggests that marital stress delays healing and increases the body's production of pro-inflammatory cytokines that can accelerate a range of age-related diseases, such as heart disease. Depressing life events, such as divorce or the death of a loved one, can even create enough stress to interfere with the heart's pump, causing "broken heart syndrome," a temporary heart failure that can lead to death if not treated.

People are more susceptible to illness when under stress, including young students who create fewer antibodies to the flu vaccine around exam time. When the reasons for patients' visits to physicians are examined, between sixty and ninety percent of visits are related to stress and other psychosocial factors. In my own practice, I've discovered that a ten-minute "stress survey" is an important diagnostic tool. Physicians need to integrate stress evaluations into standard history-taking and examinations.

America's advanced technical society is responsible for much of the information overload that causes stress, and generalized anxiety will affect all adults to some degree at different points in their life. The constant influx of information from mass communication systems such as blogging, video teleconferencing, mobile phones, email, snail mail, text messaging, instant messaging, landlines, advertisements, telemarketers, and voicemail, and the information output from the Internet, newspapers, magazines, newsletters, billboards, satellite television, and radio, causes a certain degree of information angst in everyone. Consider life in America only one hundred years ago: Only eight percent of homes had a telephone, there were eight thousand cars on the road, the speed limit was ten miles per hour, and there were only 144 miles of paved roads. Today the information highway connects people across the planet, opening the door not just to neighboring countries' cultural nuances, but to the complex socio-economic realities of second- and third-world countries which seemed remote, but the impact of 9/11 will forever remind us that the world is in our backyard. Our hearts and minds haven't caught up with technology's great lurch forward.

Stress levels rise for different reasons and in different seasons, around national holidays and periods of economic instability and recession. Post-9/11, a nationwide survey published in the *NEJM* found that ninety percent of American adults experienced a stress-related symptom. Following an economic recession, the Department of Health, Education, and Infectious Disease Center in Atlanta revealed nationwide increases in ulcers, heart attacks, impotency, weight loss, and depression. People may want to consider heading to the tanning booth the next time they're feeling in a funk. Light therapy and even tanning booths have been shown to raise serotonin levels in the organ of the skin, and can help people who suffer from seasonal affective disorder.

Job stress is one of the most universal and chronic kinds of stress. Technically, job stress is "lack of harmony between the individual and his or her work environment." Employment losses are often followed by an increase in heart attacks, hypertension, ulcers, and other pain-related illnesses and even death. Factory work and jet lag are known to create discordance between natural body rhythms and daily activities, resulting in disordered sleep patterns, mood disorders, and other medical problems. In factory work, the risk of accidental injury is significantly increased during the night shift. Perhaps more disturbing is a recent report showing that destruction of the brain's master clock rendered mice more susceptible to experimentally induced cancers.

The American idolization of youth in media such as film and television and marketing or advertisements also creates a kind of unconscious stress. In contrast to many Eastern countries such as China and Japan, older Americans are unsupported by family members, who are often scattered all over the country or overwhelmed with their immediate responsibilities. Foreigners often criticize Americans for consigning the aged and disabled to nursing homes or senior citizen communities, a concept that doesn't exist in most countries.

Time pressured-activity is another common cause of stress. The Earth moves on a twenty-four-hour cycle and so do we. Our body clocks synchronize us to our environment, and even to the seasons' changing day lengths. For this we can thank circadian rhythms, temporal programs of around twenty-four hours found in virtually all living things. Their most obvious signature is our sleep-wake cycles. But research on a wide range of organisms is revealing many clocks, working at levels from the cellular to the whole animal. The body's main circadian pacemaker is found deep within the brain's hypothalamus, which receives direct input from the retina. A recently discovered class of photoreceptors not involved in image generation contains a light-sensitive pigment. Even blind people lacking functional vision can respond to light signals with the retina's photoreceptors. The brain's "master clock" orchestrates a wide range of neural and hormonal signals, which drive a multitude of cyclical responses around the body, making routine sleep a critical component of rejuvenation and wellness.

Adding to stress is the fact that participation in organized religion has waned drastically in modern Western society, leaving people stranded in a materialistic society with no clear belief system. A general feeling of incompleteness or a spiritual vacuum haunts many people today, promoting a degree of confusion in values. The popular spiritual debate between scientists and people of faith may make some people feel like they have to choose sides: the cold, fact-filled universe of biological evolution, or the supernatural world of miracles and faith. St. Augustine, one of the greatest Western thinkers, warns against a narrow perspective of the creation story in Genesis. In my opinion, the human spirit requires neither religion nor reliance on miracles; the inherent quality or particularity to the human condition is the result of wondrous adaptive biological mechanisms that protect, sustain, and perpetuate our existence.

Acute Manifestations of Stress

Everyone has a story related to stress. My most notable one is about Scott, once a globetrotting, Google-clicking, dot-com executive. Scott headed the nuts and bolts of developing an online service in China, which was not an easy feat when people consider Beijing's obsession with controlling free speech over an Internet spanning half a billion users. Scott had been flying back and forth to Asia to carve out the terms of a multimillion-dollar deal with China's largest PC manufacturer. Two weeks spent in the purple pollution haze of Beijing would send most people to the hospital, but Scott went about his business and rushed home in time for a wedding. Upon arriving stateside after the fourteen-hour flight, his back began to itch. When he took off his shirt and asked his wife to look at the rash, a copy of the consumer edition of the *Merck Manual* in hand, she diagnosed him with shingles. The varicella zoster virus, the same virus that causes chickenpox, causes shingles. After people have had chickenpox, the virus lies dormant in one's nerves. Years later, the virus may reactivate under stress. A week later, Scott woke up with a fever, stiff neck, and the worst headache of his life. His wife left a bridal shower to take him to the emergency room, where he was evaluated for meningitis, an infection and inflammation of the membranes (meninges) and cerebrospinal fluid surrounding one's brain and spinal cord. Meningitis is a rare complication of shingles.

When I arrived at the hospital, I found Scott lying in the dark on a gurney with a bucket beside his head. He was overcome by pain so severe that he vomited continuously, making a spinal

tap to confirm the diagnosis "difficult." After Scott tested positive for viral meningitis (bacterial meningitis can progress to widespread infection of the nervous system, leading to shock and death within days), I ordered an IV with the antiviral medication valacyclovir and morphine. Complications of meningitis include permanent hearing loss, blindness, loss of speech, and brain damage leading to paralysis or even death.

Shingles is rare for people under fifty years old. People are more susceptible to shingles if they have cancer or a weakened immune system. I asked Scott's wife, a thin woman with a tall forehead and large blue eyes, if he was under a lot of stress. She told me that day in and day out for months, Scott had bowed to business demands in more ways than one. He was making the fourteen-hour flight from Washington, DC, to Beijing so often that he had earned the prestigious thousand-mile status in mileage awards. His cell phone, computer, and Blackberry buzzed late in the evening and early in the morning because of the twelve-hour time difference in business hours. She said she could often hear Scott raising his voice and repeating himself on nightly conference calls in their library, irritated with translators who often botched key terms in English, resulting in confusion and delays.

After a week in the hospital and several weeks of in-home nursing care, Scott recovered fully. Because I was concerned that he might have brushed up against a rare disease from a region famous for breeding deadly pandemics, I referred him to an "international" epidemiologist for a battery of tests. His blood work was one hundred percent normal, implying that his shingles had been triggered by stress.

As Scott's story illustrates, stress is the body's perception of a physical or psychological threat and being ill-prepared for it. The "fight or flight" response results in the body's release of stress hormones, adrenaline or noradrenaline. The short-term impact of stress includes increased metabolic, heart, and breathing rates. The long-term chronic impact can be a weakened immune system, cardiac arrhythmias, hypertension, abdominal cramping and diarrhea, and muscle tension. Inflammatory diseases that are shown to be associated with an abrupt stress response are rheumatoid arthritis, lupus, dermatitis, and asthma.

Healing Stress-Related Illness

Attitudes learned through cultural, religious, and family experiences strongly influence the way people adapt to stress. Everyone has a highly complex set of beliefs and attitudes. Each one of us sees things, including stress, in a totally different way.

Current pharmaceutical and surgical approaches cannot adequately treat stress-related illness. Holistic mind-body approaches, including nutrition, exercise, and motivating patients to change their belief structures, can help people better cope with the endemic stress of our culture. Most adults operate on a level of necessary and tolerable stress to improve performance. However, excessive long-term stress reaction can lead to illness and disease or nonphysical pain syndromes. Our physiology wasn't created or didn't evolve fast enough to cope with the burden of the kind of repeated stress and anxiety prevalent today. Emotions affect which details we remember. And things that trigger strong emotional responses, like stressful car accidents or violent images on television, are recalled more readily, according to renowned psychologist Kevin Ochsner. Ochsner's research at Columbia University examines the psychological and neural processes involved in extracting emotional and cognitive meaning from the world. His research interests include the psychological and neural processes involved in emotion, pain, and selfhood using neuroscience methods such as fMRI and the study of brain lesion populations. Perhaps one of the most valuable findings of his research is that when we're experiencing something disturbing, our brains record more details than if we were experiencing something relaxing or pleasurable.

Over a century ago, Freud proposed that people could exclude unwanted memories from awareness, a process called "repression." It was unknown, however, how repression occurs in the brain. Oschner's team used fMRI to identify the neural systems involved in keeping unwanted memories out of awareness. Controlling unwanted memories was associated with increased prefrontal activation, reduced activation of the hippocampus, and impaired retention of those memories, confirming the existence of an active forgetting process and establishing a neurobiological model for guiding inquiry into motivated forgetting. This provides a psychological model for the voluntary form of repression (suppression) proposed by Freud.

One theory for stress-related illness is that it results from repression of stress or stress-related memories. That is, part of our brain wants to react while another part tries to restrain, which results in tension. The thinking part of one's brain—the prefrontal lobes located in the front part of the brain—doesn't allow people to scream out. (Think of Edvard Munch's painting *The Scream*). The amygdala would have us screaming and jumping from tree to tree. A lot of one's negative thoughts and emotions about stress are stored in the subconscious, the unconscious part of one's mind where memories, feelings, or thoughts influence one's behavior without one's awareness. This is the key when dealing with stress-related illnesses. According to John Sarno, MD, our brains try to shove any threatening emotions into our unconscious so we don't have to become aware of them. When the feelings aren't all that intense or threatening, our brains manage to keep them repressed. However, when the emotions are particularly strong, it's harder to keep them tucked away, so the brain needs to create a distraction. It creates real physiological changes in the body, which in turn create real symptoms. These symptoms are painful or distressing enough to take one's attention away from the threatening, unacceptable feelings.

Prolonged stress and the conditioned impulse to restrain negative emotions like anger or frustration can produce incremental changes in the brain and immune system over many years. Emotional tension related to repression of negative memories, emotion, and stress contributes to the majority of pain-related, psychogenic illness—the symptoms become a distraction from the original stimulus.

Stress-provoking images, sounds and situations can cause people (especially children) to overproduce stress hormones, including the adrenal hormone cortisol, which is responsible for much of the physical damage caused by long-term stress. Chronic elevations of stress hormones contribute to a host of illnesses, including asthma, gastric ulcers, and cardiovascular disease. Children who are shy or inhibited in unfamiliar situations have been shown to suffer from multiple allergic disorders. Some of the most disturbing research on stress is showing that persistent elevations of cortisol increase the vulnerability of neurons in the hippocampus, the region that influences motivation, memory, and emotion, to damage by other substances.

The body's stress response operates autonomously but can be conditioned through the techniques we discuss in Part IV. To better understand the mechanics of stress, one will need to gain a few simple insights about the brain's multitasking functionality and the body's process of activating the stress response.

Mapping Stress

Stress starts with a perceived threat, the root of all fear, which causes the body's fight-or-flight response. The adrenal glands send adrenaline, noradrenaline, and cortisol into the bloodstream, quickening the heartbeat and raising blood pressure. The sympathetic nervous system helps redirect blood to the muscles, constricting arteries and reducing blood flow to the internal organs. Fat cells are released into the bloodstream for quick energy, not all of which are reabsorbed. The release of stress hormones makes blood platelets stickier, which might lead to the accumulation of plaque. This process occurs over and over in people who are easily stressed. But in the chronically angry, the damage is amplified because the response itself is sharper. Using a "hostility questionnaire" and angiograms, researchers have found that most hostile men have more severe arteriosclerosis.

Researchers at the University of Miami recently found that HIV-positive people who took part in stress management workshops showed improved endocrine and immune functions.

Specific brain and body regions process fear, emotions, and the physiological stress response. The brain is divided into the cerebrum, diencephalons, brain stem, and cerebellum. Three interconnection brain regions regulate fear: the prefrontal cortex, the amygdala, and the hypothalamus. The frontal lobes of the cerebrum, including the prefrontal cortex, make up sixty percent of the brain hemispheres and extend from the back of the eyes to the middle of the ears. The prefrontal cortex interprets sensory stimuli and evaluates potential danger. The frontal lobes are the "executive planning center" of the brain, enabling us to calculate, coordinate, and plan. When trauma or disease affects the frontal lobes we may become apathetic, lethargic, and unable to start or complete new tasks. Some of us may become uninhibited and start gambling impulsively and recklessly, becoming obsessed sexually and picking fights.

The second region involved in fear and aggression is the amygdala, an almond-shaped region in the limbic system (limbic means border). The limbic system borders the cortex (upper part of the brain) and the subcortex (lower part of the brain). The amygdala performs a primary role in the processing and memory of emotional reactions. Infants are born with a well-developed amygdala, which is why a baby cries when picked up by an unfamiliar person or taken to an unfamiliar place. Fear is a primitive survival tactic. Autistics have a highly reduced amygdala; they are unable to process several emotions, including the comprehension of fear or aggression in people's faces or behavioral expressions. The lack of inhibition and stimulus-seeking behavior associated with attention deficit hyperactivity disorder also may be due to disrupted connections between the amygdala and frontal cortex. The amygdala is key to intuition. Neuroscientists think that the amygdala reacts without input from the thinking part of the brain. "An emotional reaction like fear can more easily gain control over the cortex and influence cortical processes than the cortex can gain control over the amygdala." During a stressful event, the amygdala sends impulses to the hypothalamus for activation of the sympathetic nervous system and other important brain regions for increased reflexes, facial expressions, and activation of dopamine and adrenaline hormones.

Sometimes emotions can be triggered without the cortex knowing exactly what's going on. Neuroscientists refer to these emotional explosions as "neural hijackings." A key emotional area deep in the center of the brain—once again, the amygdala—proclaims an emergency, recruiting the rest of the mind and body to act. The hijacking occurs in an instant, overriding the thinking or judging part of the brain, the neocortex. Today, one in twenty Americans may be susceptible to repeated, uncontrollable emotional outbursts in which they lash out in physical abuse, road rage, or other unjustifiably violent actions. Scientists at Harvard and the University of Chicago say that neural hijackings are on the rise, and substance abuse is a typically a complicating factor. In some people with mental disorders, this may be especially strong, so their emotions are being triggered in ways that prevent them from having insight into what they are doing.

Fear follows two simultaneous paths in the brain: 1) the *unconscious*, intuitive recognition of danger flashes in the amygdala, and 2) the *conscious* executive decision making that takes place in the prefrontal cortex. The amygdala also performs primary roles in the formation and storage of detailed memories associated with emotional events. Military members in the Middle East have to be alert for surprise attacks any place, any time. This emotional and psychological conditioning can have lasting effects. For example, after the Afghan war, one of my friends said that the long, drooping clusters of Spanish moss on the live oak trees in his backyard became ominous; they were ideal perches with camouflage for snipers. He removed the long, grayish green filaments of moss. Studies on post-traumatic stress disorder connect an overabundance of fear memories in the amygdala with an inability to consciously discriminate danger from harmless phenomena.

The centrally located diencephalons in the brain include the thalamus, hypothalamus, and epithalamus. The thalamus is about eighty percent of the diencephalons, and serves as a critical relay station for sensory impulses, except for the sense of smell. The thalamus receives visual information from the eyes, auditory information from the ears, and sensory information from the body. It processes and analyzes this information and then relays it for further processing. The hypothalamus is a small region below the thalamus. The main function of the hypothalamus is homeostasis, or maintaining the body's status quo. Factors such as blood pressure, body temperature, fluid and electrolyte balance, and body weight are held to a precise value called the set point. Although this set point can migrate over time, from day to day it is remarkably fixed. Many doctors still believe the hypothalamus is the chief center governing the emotional aspect of human life. More current research supports the interaction of the brain's structures, neuropeptides, hormones, and neurotransmitters to create the chemical, electrical, and physiologic state of the living organism. There can be differences of opinion about this, but most neurologists and neurosurgeons, as well as the rest of the medical community, still do not appreciate the great influence of neuropeptides on the body.

A substantial portion of human cellular machinery is dedicated to maintaining homeostasis. In response to stress signals from the amygdala, the hypothalamus secretes corticotrophin-releasing hormone (CRH). This is a key hormone shared by the central nervous system and immune system, uniting the stress and immune responses. CRH triggers the pituitary gland to secrete adrenocorticotropic hormone (ACTH), which in turn spurs the adrenal gland to produce cortisol. Cortisol is a steroid hormone that helps people meets the demands of stress. It's also a potent anti-inflammatory agent, playing a critical role in preventing the immune system from damaging tissues. Cortisol is essential, so its levels in the blood are closely controlled. When cortisol levels rise, ACTH levels normally fall. When cortisol levels fall, ACTH levels normally rise. The body's response to cortisol is to increase blood pressure and to decrease the pulse rate. Other internal changes include a decrease in the number of white blood cells and an increase in the rate that amino acids (protein) change into sugar (glucose). CRH and cortisol are two important keys to the mind body connection.

CRH-secreting neurons of the hypothalamus regulate the autonomic nervous center (ANS), as well as the "locus ceruleus," an area of the brain stem involved in arousal, fear, and enhanced vigilance. The ANS is an entire little brain unto itself; its name comes from "autonomous," and it runs bodily functions without our awareness or control, although we can consciously alter it through techniques such as focus, meditation, and breathing exercises. The ANS includes two systems that often oppose each other: the sympathetic and parasympathetic systems. The parasympathetic system has many specific functions, including slowing the heart, constricting the pupils, stimulating the gut and salivary glands, and other responses that are not a priority when a person is threatened by danger. The body's parasympathetic system, or the "relaxation response," can be solicited through soothing music, laughter, nature, deep breathing, and other inexpensive, nonpharmaceutical techniques. The sympathetic system evokes responses characteristic of the fight-or-flight response when pupils dilate, muscles tense, heart rate increases, and the digestive system is put on hold. It also stimulates immune organs, such as the spleen.

Our knowledge about how the brain processes emotion has been gleaned through the study of the stress response. Here's a "play by play" of a familiar scene to provide a glimpse into a person's internal disaster response team. A man is driving and talking on his cell phone. The right parietal lobes of his brain are helping judge spatial relationships, and the frontal lobe provides judgment and decision making. His conscience (somewhere in the neocortex) prevents him from driving like a maniac. Suddenly, the car in front of him swerves and a two-hundred-pound buck appears in the middle of the road, antlers and all. When confronting a frightening "no eye contact" situation, animals freeze, remaining completely still for prolonged periods. Inhibiting motion reduces the likelihood of attack (except in this case, the "attacker" is a two-ton SUV barreling down the highway at sixty miles per hour). At the sight of the deer, nerves from the man's retina transmit sensory data to the visual thalamus, then the cortex and amygdala deep within the limbic system. Interactions in the cortex occur in milliseconds. Memories about death and the potential damage from hitting a deer register from the amygdala. Lightning-fast motor reflexes such as dropping the phone and clutching the wheel happen simultaneously. Meanwhile a cascade of biochemical events in the limbic system lead to the release of cortisol and chemical messengers that travel to the lower region of the brain and throughout the body. The driver begins to sweat, feel palpitations, and breathe rapidly, and if someone took a picture of his face, it would show that his expression was as frozen as the deer in the headlights.

The activity in the prefrontal lobes, just behind the forehead, takes place in microseconds. The stress response takes seconds or minutes longer because of the long road it travels throughout the body. The feeling of a near-accident stays alive in people for years. Memories are the brain's storehouses of information, both learned and significant emotional events like near-accidents. In order to create memories, nerve cells are thought to form new protein molecules and new interconnections. No one region of the brain stores all memories because the storage site depends on the type of memory—information like how to drive a car is a memory held in motor areas, while memories about smell are held in the olfactory area of the brain. The hippocampus helps the brain select where important memories will be stored. The creation of long-term memories requires attention, repetition, and associative ideas to promote new neural (synaptic) connections, such as those that are formed when practicing a sport or musical instrument. In fact, greater emotional arousal following a learning event enhances a person's retention of that event.

From an evolutionary perspective, stressful memories are stored in the brain on a subconscious level as a throwback to the ancient days when recording details of dangerous events—an encounter with a tiger or snake, for example—would lead to better ways of handling such threats in the future. One's subconscious mind (one's sleeping friend or enemy) has great influence over one's body. Touch someone, and many times they will have a flashback to a past event in their life. That's because memory is stored in the nerve cells of one's body, not just one's brain.

As we have seen, one's brain and immune system are linked at a biochemical level, continuously signaling each other through the central nervous and immune systems. One's brain interprets the cellular production of emotions, sending this information to the "thinking" part of the brain. Cognition is our ability to process and store information about the world. We are not necessarily conscious of those activities as they occur. As we saw in the example of the near-accident with the deer, many aspects of emotion rely on cognition, and cognition similarly depends on emotion.

In summary, the brain can influence the body, and the body can influence the brain. Scientists discovered that opiate receptors are all over the body and are especially dense in the brain, CNS, spinal cord, ANS, lungs, and abdomen. Heavy concentrations of neuropeptides live in the GI tract, skin, and muscles, including the heart. More amazingly, one's own white blood cells—monocytes—manufacture neuropeptides. The monocytes speak to opiate receptors in the brain, and the brain's neuropeptides speak to the body—the bloodstream, heart, lungs, GI tract, urinary system, sex organs, muscles, etc. The brain has an associative network throughout the body. When people think negative thoughts, they experience negative emotions and physiological responses like the stress response. Think fear, feel fear. Emotions are biological products of the nervous system.

The Mind-Body Connection: Holistic Medicine

Whatever people want to call it is okay with me, but I prefer "the mind-body connection." It says what it is and teaches us what we need to do. Reconnect the mind to the body. It's been centuries since Descartes decapitated us in 1630 and gave the body to science, and we still have not reconnected the brain to the body. We are graduating engineers from medical school, not holistic physicians. I'm talking about Western medicine in general. The Chinese, Japanese, and Indians got it right and have been using holistic approaches for five thousand years. The tao, "the way," the "prana"—these are all terms for the essence, the energy, and the spirit of health. These concepts have worked very well for them and still do.

I feel every pain center should have a strong mind-body connection and should use the twenty or more mind-body modalities I'll be speaking about in the next few pages. They are not addictive, cost very little, and essentially have no complications. They may not pay as much as an injection, narcotic refills, facet injections, morphine pumps, and pain-modulating implants. Pain clinics clearly make enough money from these other procedures, rather than use safer, less expensive methods which could eliminate life-threatening drug addiction and ruined lives. Today pain centers run the most lucrative business in medicine, so no excuses—after all, we are doctors and should be healers.

Holistic modalities are so numerous I can't name them all, but I will discuss the main ones. I'll include some references so people can read about others. Holistic methods should be tried first, not last. A chronic pain book by Dr. Snyder lists holistic methods, but in the back of the book, not the front. Yet this is not alternative medicine, it's mainstream medicine. Total wellness, not just pain control, should be one's goal. Read the book *The Secret of Motivating to Wellness* by Dr. Kachmann. There are many holistic treatments without medication for chronic pain problems. They are nonaddictive and work fifty to one hundred percent of the time.

Endorphins

Dr. Candace Pert wrote a famous book called *Molecules of Emotion* in which she describes the opiate receptor sites, the first time it was ever demonstrated where the chemicals in our body work. She should have received the Nobel Prize for that. A famous Scottish team used her work to discover endorphins, natural pain-relieving molecules that act like the body's own morphine. Endorphins may explain how the body is able to turn off pain sensations when it's appropriate for it to do so. Endorphins were first identified in 1975 by researchers interested in discovering how morphine works. Then they realized, to their surprise, that we make it ourselves. Dr. Pert discovered that the body had specific morphine receptors on cell membranes, chemically designed to receive only morphine. In other words, the chemical is a key that unlocks the door to the function of that specific cell. These receptors are highly concentrated in the brainstem, especially around the aqueduct of Silvius, which has spinal fluid running through it and is part of the spinal fluid circuitry system. It is surrounded by a high concentration of endorphins. Breathing techniques can stimulate them. Scientists have actually isolated at least seven different natural painkilling substances. Collectively, they make up the endorphin family.

Lamaze, a breathing technique used by women during childbirth, works because the hyperventilation causes the secretion of endorphins and relieves labor pain. It has worked for centuries and patients continue to use it today, especially in the Third World. There is growing evidence that some of the holistic methods of healing work because they release the body's natural painkillers, endorphins. Endorphins, for instance, may hold the secret to how acupuncture works. It certainly explains how meditation, yoga, tai chi, and breathing techniques in general work. It may also be the way prayer or positive thinking work. It has been found that in major war injuries, through the evolutionary mechanisms of survival, endorphins have a powerful effect and have saved many lives. If the body can naturally secrete its own pain reliever, which it apparently can, then the primary task of any person who hurts is to maximize that ability to secrete endorphins because doing so is safe and free. Endorphins work by activating the opioid receptors on nerve cells, reducing pain and lifting mood. They may also block neurotransmitters involved in communicating pain. A rush of relief and joy can trigger the release of endorphins. It's well known, for example, that people who are in the state of ecstasy simply don't feel pain the way the rest of us do. They are too absorbed in their own happiness to be bothered with pain, but also because their brain and brain stems are releasing endorphins which block the pain signal in the spinal cord. More moderate mental states, such as serenity, exercise, or engagement in a pleasing activity can result in endorphins' release.

In fact, when one's body is working properly, almost all pain signals are inhibited at least a little bit by endorphins. From minor injuries to major injuries, endorphins play a part. Certain factors can inhibit endorphins, such as anxiety, depression, and anger, all of which can result from pain. This keeps people from getting the maximum relief their bodies can provide. The pain builds on itself, leading to behaviors and mental states that increase suffering. Happily, there are many therapies available to help people stimulate endorphin production, even if the nervous system has worn out. I like yoga for its combination of physical motion and stress reduction. This really gets one's endorphins going. But a brisk walk in the fresh air can also do wonders. Massage, acupuncture, acupressure, and reflexology are also good choices. People might be surprised to hear that one of the best ways to produce endorphins is to get absorbed in a good story. Many people can temporarily block out the worst pain of a flare-up by reading, singing a song, or even watching a Hitchcock thriller, which worked for Norm Cousins, who writes about the experience in *Anatomy of an Illness*.

Guided Imagery for Pain

By creating and utilizing personal mental images, guided imagery enhances an individual's ability to make contact within the deepest level of the body, the psyche, and the soul. Guided imagery is the language of the subconscious mind. It is a way to communicate to the unconscious without thinking, in pictures. When properly programmed, the images are able to mobilize the body's intrinsic forces to heal itself. As Dr. Herbert Benson said, "There lives a doctor within us." We need to wake him up.

Guided imagery does not require a trancelike state like hypnosis does. Instead it utilizes the patient's images as the focus of activity. Visual imagery has been used for centuries. People start in a relaxed meditative state and employ breathing techniques and mind-energy mantras to quiet the mind. They visualize what they would like to accomplish and form a picture or visualization, or even make a movie in their minds. They move the pain to another part of the body, or let it escape from the body altogether. Dr. Carl Simonton teaches visualization techniques to treat cancer patients: a Pac-Man comes in and eats up the cancer cells, or bullets hit the tumor and destroy it. There are many great stories in Dr. Simonton's book *Getting Well Again*. If people visualize their pain as a fire, they can then visualize firemen all dressed up in their uniforms, dousing the flames with chemicals. The visualization should be done for a few minutes three times a day for a week or two. The activity should be preceded by deep breathing and a meditative state, followed by the visualization of the fire being doused.

Another technique is used after people are in a meditative state. They visualize a healer into their life discussing the pain and giving them advice through many different mind-body techniques in order to get this pain monkey off their back.

Visualization for Pain Relief

Find a quiet, comfortable spot where you won't be interrupted. Close your eyes and breathe quietly for a few moments. Once you're feeling relaxed, direct your attention to your pain. Note the location of the sensation, its intensity, and its precise quantities. Now, describe the pain to yourself in terms of color. Is it purple? Black? Green with yellow spots? Stay with that image for a moment, and imagine the area of your pain suffused with that color.

Now find a different color, one that has the power to dissolve or melt the color of your pain. White or silver might be a good choice. Visualize that color pouring into the painful area, dissolving the pain. You have an unlimited supply of the second color, so use however much you need. Dump buckets of it onto your pain, fuel fire hoses with it. Let rivers of the color flood your pain, washing it away. Try to spend at least five minutes with this visualization daily, preferably three times a day until the pain is gone and you can kiss it goodbye.

Holistic Therapy: Exercise

Learn the dance of life. All types of dance are great. I'm speaking about accommodation of rhythm and movement to improve longevity and intelligence. People have to use the mind to dance correctly. Ballroom dancing improves the mind and the body. Join a class and do this one or two days a week regularly. Whenever people are moving in rhythm, whether or not music is playing, they can consider themselves to be dancing. The dances of walking, jogging, biking, swimming, hiking, and even golf or tennis all follow a rhythm. Keeping in rhythm means attending to the timing of the golf swing, say, shot after shot, so that consistency is developed. I play a lot of tennis, have all my life, and really it's a form of dancing.

The effect of exercise on the immune system has been scientifically proven. Scientists have found that exercise has a direct effect on our white blood cells, the main cells affecting our immunity. Scientific studies have proven that after a few months of exercise, the levels of immune-activating cytokines produced by white cells drop over fifty percent, while the levels of immune-protective cytokines rise about thirty five percent. Exercise is probably the single most effective way to lower inflammatory factors in the blood that cause cancer and vascular disease and pain.

When physical activity is done through rhythm, it can be considered dance, and it is a powerful way to get the most benefit from one's exercise program. Pilates is an excellent, for example, as well as all other basic yoga activities. Chi-gong, tai chi, kundalini yoga, and dancing have the greatest effect on CRP (C-reactive protein) levels, the inflammatory factors in one's blood. Researchers have found that physical activity is the greatest weapon against anxiety and depression, one which has benefitted people who perform exercises such as jogging, swimming, cycling, and walking.

Adding music to rehabilitation and physical therapy programs for Parkinson's disease patients has also been shown to improve outcomes when compared to standard physical exercises. Any rhythmic movement certainly increases the level of enjoyment and involvement in exercise classes. The addition of pumping, rhythmic music to aerobic exercise classes encourages participation and increases satisfaction levels. I own a yoga studio, and I can tell you it works for our clients and us. Turning a standard exercise routine into a dance is more fun, less boring, and ensures that exercise is kept at the maximum activity level.

Why does rhythmic exercise work so much better? The answer is that rhythmic contraction, alternating between flexion and extension, provides balance and strengthens both flexors and extensors equally. The nerve impulses that regulate muscle groups originate from signals in the brain and are transmitted along the spinal cord. The same neurotransmitter chemicals released by the brain and nerve endings are sensed by our immune system. When the brain is dancing, so is the immune system. Human life itself consists of rhythms; it's quite possible that the immune system responds to these rhythms.

The concept of rhythm is an integral part of life and is as old as history. Look at the old religions, tribal dancing, Hinduism. Dancing is thought to be the arum of the universe. In Hinduism, people speak of the ancient cosmic dance of Shiva, and the frequency and randomness of all such sounds are considered to hold healing powers, as is the vocalization "ohm." Apollo, the son of Zeus and the god of medicine, was known as a dancer. In Sparta, authorities required parents to instruct their children in the art of dancing beginning at the age of five. Dancing is thought to be good for the body and overall health, as well as for the soul. Moving to modern science, researchers have shown that rhythmic music produces measurable healing effects. Music has been proven to reduce stress, pain, and anxiety, as evidenced by studies of heart patients who underwent catheterization and other unpleasant procedures. These patients' anxiety levels were significantly reduced when music was played during cardiac catheterization. People forget about their pain when music is played.

The brain uses rhythm to heal. It is important to breathe in rhythm because it affects our immunity. Healers across many different cultures have employed dance to induce a trance as part of a healing ritual. The Chinese discipline known as tai chi, which originated more than eight centuries ago, is still used as a healing art. Tai chi creates a meditative state that is set to restore natural rhythms and balance in the mind and the body. When people combine movement with rhythm, they enjoy the double benefit of exercise and the meditative state; they lower the inflammatory factors in the blood. When people have a bit of lower back pain they can benefit from rhythmic movement, even lying in bed.

Examples of rhythmic movement include:

- A thirty-minute walk every day, in rhythm

- Swimming

- Entry-level aerobics, advancing over time

- Ballroom dancing—I did it for two years with two Russian dancers

- Biking

- Rowing

- Jogging

- Jumping rope

- Tap, hip-hop, and square-dancing

- Competitive sports

- Martial arts

I recommend getting a personal trainer when possible, and starting a weight-training program.

Exercise Enhances Your Brain, Longevity and Reduces Pain

We need to go back into our evolutionary history to demonstrate the relationship among brain growth, increasing intelligence, and exercise.

To survive after forest life declined, we had to start running for our food and our brains started growing. Two million years ago, *Homo erectus* had to leave those vending machines, the beautiful forests, to catch his food, sometimes traveling ten to twenty miles a day. Our more direct ancestors, *Homo sapiens*, had to run even farther. Now our ancestors had access to oceans and lakes and those beautiful omega-3s. Brains went from weighing one pound to three pounds. The human brain became the most powerful in the world under conditions where motion was a constant evolutionary stimulus. Our brains grew under the influence of physical activity.

Are the learning abilities of someone in good physical condition different from those of someone in poor physical condition? And especially, will learning improve as physical conditioning

improves? Many studies have been done, and there are great examples out there showing that when people are couch potatoes, they will not age as well physically or mentally. The fact that exercise helps brain function is based in our evolutionary history. Certainly, exercise improves cardiovascular fitness, which in turn reduces the risk for diseases like heart attacks, strokes, obesity, and cancer. A lifetime of exercise can result in a spontaneous, astonishing elevation in learning performance, compared with those who are sedentary. Exercisers outperform couch potatoes in tests that measure long-term memory, reasoning, attention, problem solving, working, fluid, and executive intelligence. Short-term memory does not appear to respond as well to physical activity as other types of memory. Certainly the degree of improvement varies from person to person.

The amount of exercise we're talking about is not that much. Brisk walking for thirty minutes a day probably is enough. People don't have to be marathon runners. The body seems to be clamoring to go back to its evolutionary history millions of years ago. In the laboratory, the gold standard appears to be aerobics, thirty minutes at a clip, three to six times a week. Exercise is good for the brain. It increases muscle mass and decreases pain.

In my experience as a neurosurgeon, a thirty- to sixty-minute brisk walk can be as good as taking a Prozac. Exercise can help anxiety, anger, and depression. The neurotransmitters serotonin, dopamine, and norepinephrine appear to be involved. Many psychiatrists now have begun adding a regimen of physical activity to the normal course of therapy.

Scientific studies have shown that fluid intelligence, the type that involves problem-solving skills, has been particularly hurt by the sedentary lifestyle. Exercise improves children as well as adults. In a study, physically fit children identified visual stimuli much faster than sedentary ones. It has also been proven among the elderly that activities involving the senses—hearing, seeing, and balance—are greatly improved by exercise.

Eating too many calories mostly produces the free radicals, those nasty electrons that damage one's brain cells and DNA. Exercise helps reduce those free radicals by increasing blood flow and bringing more oxygen to cells, eliminating the free radicals. Getting toxic electrons out is obviously a matter of access, which is why people need increased blood supply. The brain represents only about two percent of most people's body weight, but it accounts for about twenty percent of the body's total energy usage. People's brains need a lot of glucose and generate a lot of toxic waste, which also means they need a lot of oxygen-soaked blood, which people get from exercise. When people exercise, they increase blood flow across the tissues of the body. Exercise stimulates the blood vessels to create a powerful, flow-regulating molecule called nitric oxide. This molecule enlarges one's blood vessels and relaxes them, and they become bigger, increasing oxygen supply. The more people exercise, the more tissues they can feed, and the more tissues people can feed, the more toxic waste they can remove. This happens all over the body. Exercise improves the performance of most human functions.

Another brain-specific effect of exercise recently has become clear. At the molecular level, exercise also stimulates one of the brain's most powerful growth factors, BDNE (brain-derived neurotropic factor), which aids in the development of healthy brain tissue. It increases the number of neurons and neurotransmitters. It produces neural genesis, new brain cells in the brain.

Physical exercise is like the fountain of youth and revitalizes one's brain and body. The other day while I was getting a cup of coffee, a very nice fellow started talking to me. He was about my age, and he asked me when I was going to retire. I answered by saying, "The day after I die. I'm too busy to do that."

The benefits of exercise are system wide. Physical activity affects the main targets for vascular disease and diabetes, obesity, etc. It makes the muscles stronger, bones stronger, improves our balance and strength, and reduces pain. We're less likely to have a fall, which is a common cause of a lifetime in the nursing home. Exercise regulates appetite, changes the blood lipid profile, and reduces the risk for cancer and autoimmune diseases. Exercise has a lot to do with mental health. School systems of late are eliminating exercise programs, which is a major mistake, as it has been proven that exercise helps cognitive abilities. Exercise should be integrated into the school system and the workplace; it would improve performance and eliminate a lot illnesses and diseases.

Let's face it, our evolutionary history tells us that our brains were built for walking. Improve brainpower by exercising. Exercise gets blood to the brain, brings it glucose for energy and oxygen to soak up the toxic electrons that are left over. It reduces oxidative stress and improves the function of neurotransmitters. Exercising twice a week reduces one's risk of general dementia by sixty percent.

A study of Harvard graduate students indicated that a diet consisting of approximately two thousand calories, combined with exercise, positively impacts longevity and mental health. Physical activity really does matter. Aerobic exercise burns about three hundred calories a day. That means walking briskly for about forty minutes would do the job. Walking slowly would take about seventy minutes, stationary bike about thirty minutes. Exercise beyond that, some studies show, doesn't have many additional health benefits.

As you can see, a small amount of exercise—for most individuals, a brisk walk for little more than a half hour per day—will more than meet their requirements. Not surprisingly, this simple form of exercise also generates a nearly seventy percent reduction in the incidence of breast cancer in women. Moderate exercise is an exceptionally useful drug. It lowers excess blood glucose and excess insulin, since exercise requires the use of stored energy. Most of the stored energy will come from fat.

If some exercise is good, isn't more better? A more careful inspection of the longevity curve and exercise indicates that after about two thousand calories per week, the curve simply flattens out. As people increase exercise intensity, they also increase the levels of oxidative stress on the body. Remember those nasty free radicals that are due to oxidative stress on the body? Exercise requires a lot of use of oxygen, the big producer of free radicals. People who exercise more than a moderate amount are making more free radicals because their muscles require more ATP, which has its origins in food, the biggest producer of free radicals yet. Although these people will be fitter, they probably won't live longer, although Jack LaLanne would probably argue about that. The second reason excessive exercise may not be beneficial is that the more intense the exercise, the greater the production of cortisol in response to the stress. Thus, higher exercise intensity actually can increase two pillars of aging—free radicals and cortisone. If one's goal is longevity, moderate exercise is the best course of action. The more intense the exercise, the faster the oxidative candle burns, and the more free radicals people produce.

One's function later in life will, of course, improve with regular exercise. People will have stronger muscles and bones and be less likely to take a fall and experience injury. Functionality in later years will strongly depend on exercise to preserve muscular strength and for quality of life to improve.

The anti-aging benefits of exercise are mediated through different hormone systems. The first hormonal system directly affects one of our four posts of aging, excess insulin. The reduction of insulin will be achieved primarily by aerobic exercise. Aerobic exercise simply means exercising at the intensity at which sufficient oxygen is delivered to the muscle to do the required work. As people age, their aerobic capacity decreases, which means they have to lower their intensity of exercise to maintain sufficient oxygen transfer to the muscles. The longer people exercise aerobically, the more they lower the insulin level.

Exercise builds muscle mass through a growth hormone and testosterone. The secretion of these hormones will be increased by anaerobic exercise, exercise that is not as vigorous as aerobic exercise. Anaerobic exercise is any exercise whose intensity causes insufficient oxygen transfer to the muscle cells. This rapidly produces lactic acid as a breakdown product of glucose, which causes a burning sensation in the muscles.

In aerobic exercise, muscles normally take blood glucose for their increased energy needs. Actively exercising muscles take up nearly thirty percent more glucose than those at rest. This uptake of blood glucose is a noninsulin-driving event. If there is not enough glucose or glycogen available during exercise, like in a marathon run, then cortisone or stress predominates. The more effectively the glucagon system is working to maintain blood glucose level, the less the backup systems are called into play. That is why lower-intensity aerobic exercise ensures that adequate blood glucose levels are maintained for the brain, thereby keeping the backup hormonal systems of adrenaline, and especially cortisol, in reserve. The more intense the exercise, the more growth hormone and testosterone are released. This occurs about fifteen to thirty minutes after the exercise has been completed. That is why anaerobic training, light weightlifting, and wind sprints are ideally suited for maximizing new muscle mass development. People must feel the burn in the muscles to achieve this. Growth hormone release is primarily needed to repair the micro tears in the muscles that occur during intense anaerobic exercise. Unfortunately, the more insulin in the bloodstream, the fewer growth hormones are released, regardless of the intensity of anaerobic training. That means that all the hormonal benefits of anaerobic exercise can quickly be undone by a high-carbohydrate sports energy drink consumed just after exercise.

Exercise is important, but still not as important as eating the right diet. Diet can impart a far greater effect on one's anti-aging program than exercise alone. That is why people probably only need to exercise an hour per day, but remember, people can eat twenty-four hours per day. As a consequence, all the hormonal benefits of exercise may be offset by one's diet. Dr. Barry Sears likes the 80/20 rule. Eighty percent of one's health benefits will come from diet; only twenty percent will come from exercise. Using of the two together, people have a formal drug combination to lower insulin levels.

Pain Has Many Friends

Let us strip a few complex pain problems down to bare-bones, reductionist thinking.

For the beginning of this problematic way of thinking, see *Discourse on the Method of Rightly Conducting One's Reason and of Seeking Truth in the Sciences,* René Descartes.

Pain can be used as a tool to make a lot of money, we all know that. Sometimes people do this consciously, some believe the story they're telling after a while, and some are just plain fraudulent.

Pain is a friend to millions of people. They wouldn't want to give it up because they would lose that monthly check. Frankly, it's almost understandable, but is it right? Is it honest? Insurance companies even send out investigators now to videotape their customers doing heavy work at home while collecting disability payments based on a painful back. Certainly there are also many people who have a significant pain problem and cannot get Social Security or their insurance company to pay them the money they deserve. This is a complex issue.

There are probably twenty million people on Social Security disability because of pain. I personally feel that many of them could actually work but they perceive themselves as being disabled. Many have been through horrific treatment at pain centers, questionable surgeries, and been over-prescribed narcotic medications.

Unfortunately the best way to get Social Security disability for someone to say they have a painful back condition. People who work in a factory do a lot of bending and twisting. How people could possibly do that? So there is a very fine line here between truth and reality. I've been in this business for forty years and I see this fine line being crossed all the time, especially in bad economic times when people are getting laid off. That's when disability claims skyrocket. It is quite understandable that at a time like this, pain could be a friend.

X-rays, CT scans, and MRIs many times don't match the problem. Providers take advantage of that anyhow and use the studies as a nocebo, promoting injections and procedures and narcotic medications. Once providers habituate or addict the patient, they are a guaranteed returning customer who needs another prescription, maybe be for lifetime. I see this a lot in the disability game.

Eventually the neural circuitry of the brain is changed and the perception of pain never goes away. There's also a reward at the end, a settlement or monthly check. If people are desperate economically, it can lead to pain-seeking behavior. People may see this as the only way out to take care of themselves and their family, even though most disability checks are not that large.

After two years of Social Security disability people are eligibile for Medicare, and they might even be able to get food stamps. When you add all that up, especially since most of it may be tax-free, you find people who are making as much as the average American without working. Believe me, there are huge portions of the population who have figured this out.

Work-related injuries most of the time are pain-related; the great majority of time we don't find the cause for certain. Nothing is broken, and MRIs merely show the process of aging in the spine. Yet providers make something out of it, producing three-page x-ray reports with which the patient becomes obsessed, and the circle of pain treatments starts. Addictive drugs are high on the list and patients' sick leave is long. People may even get a disability rating with a pretty good-sized check when it is financially settled. In Florida, unless they recently changed the law, a person may receive workman's comp disability at his or her present wage until death. What do you think? Are some people taking advantage of that pain story? That's why we see so many pain centers: there's money there. When I see these patients as second opinions, the majority of the time I have no living idea why they hurt. I have no living idea why they received all the treatments for their complaints. Maybe multiple people are making a lot of money. Unfortunately, sometimes we have to face the truth. I generally find that these patients would be a lot better off working. Most of them are breaking up their families through these addictions and are not very happy. I find that in certain states like Ohio, the work-related back injury can turn into a lifetime affair, with no motivation to return to work. Laws vary from state to state. In Indiana there is a cutoff point; you get PPI rating and a settlement is made. People will get a check based on the rating, but unfortunately the employer may terminate them. This is listed on their work record and they may not be hired in the future because of it. Many times this is not fair to the patient. When I treat people I always consider the goal to be making them healthy enough to return to work. That is where happiness is. I'm working full time at age seventy-four, just believe me.

A disabled patient can be a lifetime customer for a pain center. Providers there periodically inject people and then habituate or addict them to drugs and the circle never ends. It's the Rolodex at work, the perfect money-making business.

As a matter of fact, once people get a settlement from workman's comp, they will continue with the pain center, and then they apply for Social Security disability and eventually get Medicare. A monetary reward indeed. Happiness is another matter.

Believe me, a job would be better psychologically for the patient and family. Many end up as drug addicts and drift into depression, anxiety, fear, and hopelessness. This is a huge problem across the country. Only three percent of the people who receive a Social Security check ever get back into the workforce. The motivation is gone. They could go back to school and learn something different to make a living, but the monetary benefits suppress the motivation to do this. Very few of these people ever get better.

Many people have a psychiatric need for pain. It's their way of life. It's how they control their families or loved ones—"I can't do this" and "I can't do that." "No sex tonight, my back hurts." Without the pain they would feel no purpose in life. They go from doctor to doctor and get a different diagnosis every time. There are tests to be run, procedures to be done—it gives them something to do. Many times a symptom switches to differ-ent parts of the body. From headaches to chest pain, back pain, or pelvic pain, there is a lot of territory to spend time on. It would be better to get involved with a wellness program and feel good again. But "the worried well," they keep the doctors busy, and if a provider decides to make some money, it can result in a lot of unnecessary procedures. I have seen hun-dreds of injections and unnecessary back surgeries on the "worried well." They go from pain center to pain center, endure multiple CDs, MRIs, and injections, and are on ten different medications. Pain is their life; if it were taken away, they might even commit suicide. They are spinning the wheel, controlling society and the family around them. The majority are anxious, depressed, and angry people. "Look at poor me, the only reason I don't achieve is because I hurt"—a very common story. The patient is one hundred percent convinced of their pain problem and I agree that it's absolutely real to them. Certainly drug habituation or addiction can make it more real because of the changes in the brain's neural circuitry.

I see a significant number of people on Social Security disability because of fibromyalgia, a treatable condition that can be healed through mind and body techniques, unless the patient is a negative thinker and this is his way of life. I would like to point out that we only live once and there might be a better way. We all have a talent for something; we need just to keep on looking.

Of course, lawsuits for minor injuries are common, and pain works best. Unfortunately, many of these patients actually convince themselves that they are severely disabled rather than suffering a minor condition, a condition I can't even demonstrate on x-rays, and many time they proceed to ruin their lives. Certainly some of them carry out a conscious fraud and then sail off into the sunset when they get the check, but in my experience this takes three to five years. That's a lot of life to give up, and it can never be recovered. A person's way of thinking may have changed in that time and his spouse may not be living with him anymore, as "we can't do this or that because my back hurts" doesn't go very far with the spouse who knows the real story. Insurance companies are making big mistakes. They should quickly settle cases with some cash in their hands, and I would walk into the house with a wad of cash and try to settle the case. Within a month of an accident that results in minor injuries, most people are desperate for a little bit of money instead of dragging it out forever. Many times these patients receive unnecessary injections, medications, and procedures, all of which could be avoided, saving the insurance company a lot of money. It would keep our insurance rates low. I've been in this business for forty-one years but the insurance companies never change. They give people such a hard time that they need to go to court and a lawyer instead of settling for bit less a lot sooner. Many times, while waiting for the insurance company's decision, patients convince themselves they are probably disabled and have to leave the workforce. The insurance settlements generally are not large enough to sustain them for the rest of the lives and their family may be economically ruined.

As usual the providers at pain centers have a ball in situations like these. Everybody is making money because the treatment bills are huge. Many providers accept that the patient can't pay the bill until a settlement occurs. I spoke to a chiropractor the other day who said that many times the patient keeps the settlement money at the end. Perhaps a just reward for unnecessary treatment.

Occasionally people accuse doctors of malpractice using faked pain or paralysis. I was reading about neurosurgeon in Florida who lost a malpractice case because of the patient's pain problem. He was persistent, though. He was able to photograph the patient's lawyer and the patient sailing through the Caribbean from island to island, securing the boat's rigging, out of his usual wheelchair. The lawyer and patient were convicted of fraud. Justice does not happen that often.

So pain can be one's friend, but most the time it ruins the people's lives. It changes a person's mental state. Leaving the workforce and giving up a useful life can put a person on the road to disability, which leads to depression, anxiety, anger, and broken families.

I've worked in the Veterans Administration system. I'm a Vietnam vet myself. I'm proud of the servicemen. Then again, the amount of pretended disability I see is almost not believable. It's nearly understandable, though: people get paid for pain, and the more pain people have, the more money people get. I constantly see patients who try to increase disability payments by using MRI scans that actually show nothing more than the natural process of aging. Many of these people are overweight, drink too much, smoke too much, and are already living joyless lives trying. They are trying to increase disability benefits based on pain. Incidentally, this is something that accompanies every war. No one ever gets well; in the VA system that would only decrease one's check. There are no awards for wellness. No check for losing fifty pounds, or for giving up alcohol or cigarettes. What does get you a check? Developing cancer or type II diabetes. Type II diabetes is curable through weight loss, but no one gets a check for that. If someone stops smoking there's no check for that, either!

Economic need is indeed a motivator. Is it fraud? We need to change the system. We should pay people for wellness, not for pain. Of course, the horrible injuries of war that result in real neuropathic pain with nerve damage should be generously compensated. Then again, the majority of the patients being treated do not fall into this category.

Lastly, I see a lot of disability games in the railroad workman's comp and retirement system. I read about a scandal in New York City railroad retirement system. They actually did call it a fraud. Just before retirement, the employee would go to a certain physician who was in on the fraud. The doctor would give the employee a high disability rating, which would be directly reflected in his lifetime pension.

So pain is a complex issue, the source of a lot of fraud and a lot of unhappiness and disability, real or not real. Pain can be one's friend and enemy.

The Difficult Patient, the Difficult Doctor, and the Difficult Pain Problem

Pain is a sensation, a cognition, an emotion. It's just not pain. The brain is attached to the human body, contrary to the belief of most; we are reattaching it, in some part of the country more than others.

To treat chronic pain takes a lot of patience, a lot of time, a loving provider, a positive way of thinking, and a teacher with a plan, such as a placebo doctor, a natural healer. I don't see a lot of these people at pain centers. I realize that treating pain is not an easy business. Physicians find fifteen percent of the pain patients difficult to deal with, which matches my experience. Truth be told, though, if doctors really talked to these people rather than just handing out prescriptions, or if they refused to give a narcotic prescription, the number of difficult patients would skyrocket. The narcotic Rolodex saves a lot of time; a doctor only needs to talk to the patient for a minute or two. I know because I talk to the patients about it. Many the pain doctors run auxiliary offices out of town—some have as many as six. I see these in TV and newspaper advertisements. Can you imagine the number of people they are addicting to drugs? These newspaper articles about narcotic-related deaths certainly give us a hint. The less empathetic the physician, the more likely he will find the patients difficult to deal with, especially he takes the time to talk to them.

About thirty to fifty percent of chronic pain patients experience some sort of psychopathology, depression, anxiety, personality disorder, or substance abuse. In her excellent book *Pain Chronicles*, Melanie Thernstrom claims, after extensive research, that the psychopathology comes on after a patient develops pain. That could mean it is due in part to undertreatment, but I predict it is much more from overtreatment, unnecessary procedures and narcotics used to attempt to treat the condition. Besides, after reading her great book, I'm not convinced that she really knows that the majority of the pain problems are from narcotic addiction and habituation, not from neuropathic pain. She always seemed to be talking about neuropathic pain, which is only a small part of the chronic pain problem. Certainly, habituation and addiction produce withdrawal symptoms, anxiety, depression, and substance abuse. That's why the patients go to the emergency room, because the pain centers and their doctor's offices are closed for refills, and the cycle continues. I don't think emergency rooms should refill prescriptions on the weekend for chronic pain patients unless they have cancer; we don't in our office. The doctor on call will not give narcotic prescriptions on Saturday or Sunday unless it's an absolute emergency.

About a month ago I had a very difficult patient admitted to me by the doctor on call. I had operated on him for a ruptured disc about five years earlier. It was work-related injury, involved with the Ohio workman's comp system, which is a fairly generous system from my point of view. Unlike in Indiana, the Ohio system seems to have no endpoint; the checks just keep on coming. It's even worse in Florida, where they pay one's normal wages for a lifetime. For the truly disabled this is a wonderful thing, but a lot of people are milking the system, sitting at home collecting the checks and never getting well. If they got well they would not get a check. A fraud?

When my patient recovered from the original ruptured disc, I sent him back to work. Unbeknownst to me, I think he claimed some back pain and his family doctor sent him to a pain center, and the ballgame began. First came the injections; they made their money, then the narcotics started, and the band played on. The pain center reduced this individual to helplessness, divorce, and eviction, and totally destroyed him. I didn't say to him, "Where do you hurt?" I said, "What's going on in your life?" It was a horror story.

Out of this complex story I did manage to figure out that he had recently lifted a couch while trying to move in with his girlfriend because he couldn't afford his own place and had developed a large recurrent ruptured disc. He clearly had a foot drop and needed surgery. I warned him that though I could resolve his foot drop, the procedure certainly would not solve his chronic pain problem. And it didn't.

For a week after the operation, it was a nightmare on the neurosurgery floor. Before the patient came in he had been on five different medications, a very difficult situation to balance postoperatively. The nurse supervisor and I each spent an hour with the patient every day; his actual floor nurse just threw in the towel. It's tough to get me excited, but I must say he was ringing my bell too. He liked me, though; in spite of everything, I got along with him. I called in an excellent psychiatrist whom I consider to be the most dedicated physician in the hospital, but he never got started with the patient. He told me the next day that he had about eight chronic pain consultations that day. That was besides the other routine psychiatric consultations. The hospital was clearly overburdening this wonderful physician who truly understands chronic pain and its psychiatric aspects. Besides me, there's no one in the city more upset about chronic pain centers and addictive drugs in general. He could really write this story himself, but in my experience it's tough to get a doctor to even write a chapter in one of my books. I would love to take advantage of his knowledge.

Eventually I was able to get this patient home, but he refused to go to the drug rehab center. Let's face it, the probably started at the pain clinic and their narcotic medications. If they had sent the patient back to me this never would have happened. I run a wellness center with all sorts of holistic modalities right in the hospital. I have to be thankful to the community health service system, Lutheran Hospital specifically, for allowing me to do that. We are getting a lot of people well there without giving narcotics, and we teach a lot of mind-body health, including classes in proper eating. I don't know what's going to happen to this patient; he did talk a little bit about some schooling available through the Ohio workman's comp, and I highly encouraged him to partake in it. He's young and intelligent and he fully realizes something needs to change; it's the addiction that's the problem. In this case I think psychiatric care probably is the answer, but the patient must be willing. There are many cases like this out there. Prevention is the key.

The Helpers and Killers: Pain Medicine

Certainly, there's a place for pain medication, anti-inflammatories, tranquilizers and antidepressants, aspirin, Tylenol, and narcotics. The problem is that we abuse them and there are too many side effects. Most of us physicians don't even know all the side effects—we are not aware of how they all interact, and we don't know how to properly prescribe them.

People might think pain centers are the answer. My experience with them, though, is that they tremendously overprescribe medications. I don't agree with their definition of pain. When the epidural blocks don't work, the spinning wheel of narcotics begins.

Some patients with neuropathic or cancer pain clearly need strong medication, including narcotics. Some will need to be on them for a lifetime, and for these people the drugs are a godsend. That doesn't mean they can't try holistic methods in addition. The concern about habituation and addiction should be minimal in this group of patients. Contrary to many pain books, I see no evidence whatsoever of doctors refusing to give narcotics to people with truly neuropathic pain or cancer. I see daily how doctors misread diagnostic tests and then generously dispense narcotics to patients experiencing metabilic pain (centralized brain pain) without clear cause. I was on call one night and received another patient with a very confusing story, but in the middle of it all was a pain center. The patient had exaggerated her symptoms in front of her husband, but I got the true picture pretty quickly—a lot of symptoms, even hysterical paralysis, and twenty MRIs in five years with no findings. Clearly metabilic pain (centralized brain pain).

In his book *Inside Chronic Pain*, Lous Heshusius says a 2005 policy analysis by the Cato Institute in Washington, DC, found that the DEA's painkiller campaign has cast a chill on the doctor-patient candor necessary for successful treatment. I don't know how wrong this person could be. I see absolutely no hesitation by physicians prescribing narcotics, especially for routine problems. He's just plain wrong. Pain treatment is not scarce; there are many doctors in the field of pain management, and they're everywhere, making a financial fortune.

The case against narcotics frankly is mainly not just habituation, addiction, and the sensitization they cause the nervous system, but that they don't work very much. They only work thirty percent of the time in thirty percent of the people—anyone doing research on pain medication knows that. It's called a 30/30 law. Almost two hundred million prescriptions for pain relief are written in the United States each year, but fewer than a third of the people on opioids report any relief. Yet these drugs are necessary for a significant number of people. The government clearly is not interfering with the medical use of narcotics for pain, believe me. What I see in the hallway in waiting rooms of pain centers is beyond human description—opium dens would be a friendly term.

There is a false assumption that painkillers are the only and best way to manage pain. Many patients and providers

don't understand the side effects of what they're prescribing or taking. Most believe that painkillers rarely kill. But the adult daughter of one of my best friends recently died from a prescription she received from a pain doctor. I've always pictured a target on the front of that doctor's chest, but I add one on his back too. He cannot continue to do what he's doing. The government so far has done nothing, although I've asked abused pain patients to send their stories to their government officials. I don't know what else I can do except maybe write a book. which I'm clearly doing.

The correct way to treat pain is not taught in medical school, and if the pain centers do the teaching, things will get even worse. There are a few excellent centers, of course, and I understand the issue is very complex. Most physicians have not even heard of the use of the nocebo, that test that has no relationship to the actual problem. This often happens in cases of degenerative disc disease. These tests do not help but rather misdirect patients. A good pain clinic, on the other hand, may prescribe pain medication, but will also discuss holistic methods of pain management, and will try them at the beginning of treatment, not the end.

Dr. Fishman wrote a famous book called *War on Pain*. It emphasizes the point that one may need to try many different type of medications to arrive at the right combination for pain relief. Trial and error is part of the treatment.

One of those pain specialists says there are at least fifty medications people could pick from. There's no way of knowing which one a patient will respond to, so this approach may have some value. It may take a year of tinkering with different medications and combinations to find the right one. I assume we're talking about neuropathic pain, because medication should not be the first choice if there has not been clear-cut nerve damage. Metabolic Pain (centralized brain pain) caused by the neurochemistry of one's brain should not be treated with narcotics, but it may respond to medications like antidepressants and tranquilizers.

Many medical providers may bail out if people don't respond quickly to treatment, so people have to be patient. Sometimes people may need a psychotherapist in addition to their family doctor, pain specialist, or holistic doctor. Pain may vary from day to day, so the treatment will have to vary accordingly. I'm not against pain medications per se— I still recommend plenty of them—but the short- or long-term adverse effects pose serious problems that people should avoid as much as possible.

People may try anti-inflammatories, opioids, muscle relaxers, anti-depressants, and anxiety drugs. Anticonvulsants are also used. Many of these have serious side effects and patients must know what they are. They can read and memorize the drug insert themselves; odds are they will know more about it than their provider. I admit it, many patients know more about their medication than I do. Remember, medication may help the pain without making it totally go away. It takes the unbearable and makes it bearable. Serious side effects of these medications can include drowsiness, agitation, rebound headaches, stomach pain, nausea, ulcers, bleeding, vomiting, serious constipation, increased depression, heightened anxiety, cognitive disturbances to the point that one can't think, hallucinations, and impaired short-term memory. Every drug has the potential to make the very thing it's trying to treat worse. People can die from the medication.

Some think morphine is the worst because of the extreme constipation it causes. That's all people need is a stomach pain on top of other pain. Laxatives may need to be taken with morphine. All opiates cause constipation. Occasionally morphine can cause hallucinations as well, especially at night. In the daytime morphine may confuse people and put them in a dense fog. Movements slow down, and people experience memory problems.

These side effects alter life in major ways. People lose the ability to attend to the relevant feedback from their bodies, resulting in a lot of problems. The side effects can produce problems that interfere with living. So the question always is, "Do I want my mind distorted and have less pain? What should I try to put up in order for my mind to stay clear?" When the pain is severe, of course, the mind cannot stay clear either. That's when I recommend the addictive medication.

The struggle with adverse effects is exhausting. I don't think most providers have any idea what it means to deliberately risk the side effects that interfere with daily living and thought processes, and increase the potential for injury through accidents and overdoses. Almost everyone, no matter his or her economic status, knows someone who died from an overdose of narcotic medication. In our surrounding counties we have seventy deaths every year due to physician-prescribed narcotics. There are probably more than fifteen thousand of these deaths in the nation. Let's face it, it's a war on pain. The taking of drugs is a huge part of the daily lives of chronic pain patients, and we need to change that. How can people trust a doctor's knowledge when it comes to drugs? They can't. And that's not because they don't trust the doctor, it's that the medications are just too unpredictable and complex, especially when they interact with other drugs. Further, many of these medications are used off label and have not even been tested by the Food and Drug Administration. Even Tylenol is a dangerous drug—frequent use, as little as 1000 mg, can cause chronic obstructive pulmonary disease and decreased lung function, and higher doses can affect the liver and kidneys, even resulting in death.

I would always try mindfulness pain reduction from the beginning. The books of Jon Kabat-Zinn, as well as his CDs, have been very helpful to many patients. I run a mindfulness course almost year-round at my Mind Body Institute in Fort Wayne, Indiana. We feature five lectures by Dr. David Johnson from the University of St. Francis and we are expanding his programs. I'm doing a DVD with him soon. Dr. Johnson is very good at teaching this course. I also recommend the books, DVDs, and CDs of Vidyamala Burch, Dr. Jackie Gardner, and Lous Heshusius.

The Legal Addict

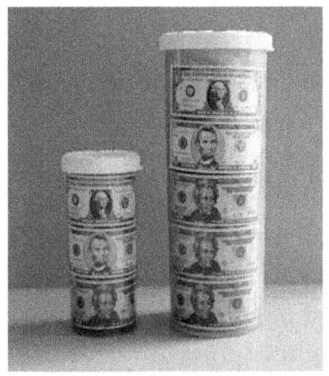

A recent national newspaper confirmed something I've known all along, and something I know the public has known too, because I had been asking my patients what they thought was the biggest cause of drug addiction in this country. The news media has finally woken up to the same realization: it's physician prescriptions. It's not the guys from Mexico and Colombia, yet who is sitting in jail? How do we stop this national scandal? Are physicians causing drug addiction?

There are now more legal addicts on the street than illegal addicts. My local newspaper is warning about this, and I wrote an editorial for them, but they never followed up with an investigative report to discover the real truth. I doubt they'll do it at this time. Maybe they are afraid of offending their paying advertisers?

I had been speaking about this problem in the doctor's lounge with another doctor. Later I saw him in the emergency room; he did not know I was sitting behind him. He had just ordered 15 mg of morphine for a patient with chronic pain of unclear etiology. The patient had told him, "You know, Doctor, I'm a legal addict." That's exactly the problem—millions of legal addicts in this country were created and maintained by the industrial complex and the medical profession. Let's open our eyes and have a real look at it. We may be undertreating an occasional acute pain and neuropathic pain, but no one will die from that. We are overtreating the other seventy percent. Certainly there are a few great pain centers in this country, where they treat the patient holistically and hand out a few medications as needed. But we must change the culture that the "gold standard" of pain treatment is the word of the patient. We have a culture of hurt; our biology, physiology, and emotions affect our perception of pain. It is very characteristic of American culture. It needs to change or we'll have a nation of habituated and addicted people. We pay money to people who have pain, and we pay the providers of pain-relieving procedures handsomely, but we don't pay much for results. They don't send disability checks to people who have no pain. No narcotic medication should be handed out to a patient unless the medical provider has a look at a national program INSPECT, which is getting better and better. It records every patient and every physician who is writing narcotic prescriptions. It takes time to look at a website, however, and an emergency room physician or office doctor would need to be paid for that time. We need to ask the patient, "What's going on in your life?" before we ask, "Where does it hurt?" Legal addicts flood the emergency room in the evenings and on weekends; they panic because their doctor's office is closed. At least if they have a personal doctor he might know something about the patient, but a number of offices exist basically to write narcotic prescriptions. Another doctor told me that. I spoke to a very thoughtful doctor in the emergency room the other day named Alex. He looked at the INSPECT site every time he had a patient who claimed to need a narcotic prescription. I'd like to give him a medal. He has also referred a few patients to my Mind Body Institute to try a holistic approach to the chronic pain.

The legal addict has a lot better chance in the emergency room because nobody knows him. Even if he gets admitted there is a good chance he will get overtreated because the nurse will institute the fifth vital sign—"What is your pain level on a scale of 0 to 10?" The doctor on call is hopelessly lost in these cases and says okay to the pain meds. Otherwise the nurse supervisor may be called, and if this happens a few times he may end up in front of a hospital committee. Lawyers have sued some health care providers for not treating pain. Judgment has become irrelevant, and that certainly has helped create an army of pain addicts.

Ninety percent of the time chronic pain is just a nuisance. It has no value but causes sleep loss, anxiety, depression, suicide, unnecessary medication, unnecessary surgery, tremendous cost, real and imagined disability, and so on. Rarely does chronic pain reveal a hidden problem like a benign tumor, though I have seen this occasionally over the years. Why did God or nature put chronic pain in the body in the first place? It is probably caused by the stress of life and modern times and is promoted by people who make money from it, everyone from the patient to the provider, the industrial complex, and the lawyers. Every war is followed by a legion of veterans seeking disability for real and imagined pain problems. "I hurt, I get paid; I don't, I get nothing." In my experience, the most common cause of a poor result from back surgery is not that the surgeon didn't do enough, it's because they operated on a patient who didn't need the surgery in the first place. Usually the human body and nature help us get better—there's a doctor who lives within us, Dr. Herb Benson would say. Unfortunately, with chronic pain, Mother Nature is fooling us. The human body is part of the chronic pain fraud. Treatments like surgeries and narcotics rarely help and have destroyed many people with the help of others.

The Two Arrows

For thousands of year, the Hindu tradition has looked at pain holistically, connecting the body and the mind. They didn't have the Cartesian reductionist way of thinking, where the head was cut off from the body, as Descartes did in 1637. To Hindus, pain is body-mind, mind-body. They use the metaphor of the two arrows. Arrow number one is a physical pain that people feel from an illness, disease, or injury. Arrow number two is the emotional reaction—one's anxiety, emotion, sensation, obsession, and pain experience. When people experience acute pain, they know what it is, where it is, and how to fix it so that the pain goes away the majority of the time. Arrow number one has been cured, unless one's health care provider continues to prescribe addictive drugs and people get hooked, building a case for arrow number two. In some pain problems, it is a choice of the individual and provider to continue with the treatments and medications, or people may have chronic pain (pain lasting more than a few months) and their brain chemistry starts playing a part in the case through emotional reactions, anxiety, fear, and anger. Resistance to the pain, framing it through negativity and not dealing with it positively, results in a bigger problem.

Patients with metabolic pain -pain based on the chemistry of one's mind, thought process, neuropeptides, hormones, and neurotransmitters) can affect the pain that is produced.

A part of the brain called the **cingulate gyrus** coordinates sensory input with emotions, produces emotional responses to pain, and regulates aggressive behavior. The cingulate gyrus does not know the difference between acute and chronic pain. So the sensation of pain or experience of pain is the same for a person. "I hurt," they say, "I have severe pain," but we can't find a clear cause. Yet it is real to the patient.

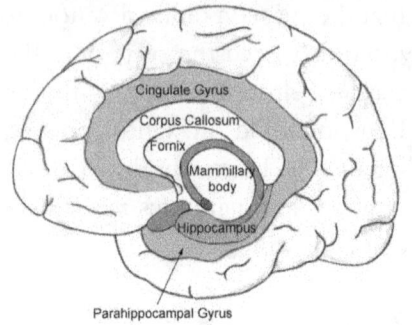

Mindful teaching is the answer. Frontal lobe lobotomies are out of style. Actually I did some during my surgical training, and the patient would say, "I have pain, but I don't feel it."

If people have only arrow two metabolic pain (pain caused by the molecules of emotion, neuropeptides, hormones, neurotransmitters, and impulses from the autonomic nervous system), they should not be treated with narcotics, injections, or surgeries. Mindful treatments are the treatments of choice. They result in no addictions or complications, and have no risk.

Vidyamala Burch's Five-Step model of Mindfulness Treatments for Chronic Pain

Step 1

Developing mindfulness about what actually is happening at the moment is the first step in chronic pain treatment, teaching more awareness of the pain itself, more awareness of one's breathing, awareness of one's surroundings, the greenness of the grass, and the blue sky. Mindfulness and meditation go together.

Step 2

Facing pain is essential because we need to see the face of chronic pain. Resisting it or drowning it has no value. We need to see the pain for what it is.

Remember, the first arrow can be treated and cured by fixing the pain and it goes away, but the second arrow produces suffering. People are either blocking pain or drowning in it. It is their own reaction. People may resist chronic pain and suffering, but they can also learn to work with the pain with awareness and using their breath to move the pain out of the brain into the body, or getting rid of it completely. People can breathe with the pain and with awareness, exhaling it with a sense of letting go. The body scan is an excellent method.

Over time people can learn to adapt a timely and nonjudgmental attitude to the whole of the experience and allow painful sensations just to be present and not bothersome. People may not be able to get rid of all the pain but they can reduce their reaction to it and not make such a big deal about it. When people bring awareness and curiosity to the actual experience of pain, they often find it is not as bad as they feared it would be. It's like quitting smoking—it's usually fear that keep people from doing it. Withdrawal symptoms are minimal, yet a lot of people have a hard time with it.

Step 3

Seeking the pleasant part of chronic pain involves becoming sensitive to the pleasant part of the expression of pain. There's always something pleasant in one's life, it just depends on how you look at it. Happiness is dependent on one's point of view. As Norman Vincent Peale said as he walked out of his hotel on a cold, icy, and snowy day in Chicago, "Isn't it just the most beautiful, god-awful day?" It depends on one's point of view. Positive thinkers appreciate the five senses as they observe their environment—what they smell, touch, and hear, the singing of the birds, the colors of the rainbow, the beauty of the family. People wishing to cultivate positive feelings can focus on the love of their family, appreciate their job no matter what it is, or spend free time watching a movie, reading, or listening to a good song. I talk to the birds, I talk to the flowers, and it sure makes me feel better no matter what my situation is that day. Music changes my mood in seconds when I'm driving home from work.

Step 4

Broaden awareness to include the pleasant and unpleasant aspects of one's pain experience. Push away from pain and into the life around you. Become a bigger container. Allow a sense of space, freedom, and stability. Become aware of other people, of the rest of the world.

Step 5

Learn to respond rather than react. Don't block the pain and overwhelm yourself. Resisting the pain only adds to the problem. Ask yourself, "Am I being overwhelmed with negative talk about my x-rays, CT, MRIs, or angiograms? Are these results really related to my problem, or am I being noceboed by my health care provider?" This occurs very frequently in pain centers. Notice your experience rather than trying to avoid it. Move toward the pain and seek out the pleasant.

The point is we need to change our relationship with pain. We need to accept it, beware of it, and reduce our resistance to it, and then it will be reduced over time. Resisting it will not help people with chronic pain. Resistance produces blocking, and overwhelming it only makes it worse. Resistance to pain is the major cause of suffering and distress. That is why people are getting pierced with the second arrow. Many people turn to distractions because of blocking and seek relief in alcohol, drugs, and addictive medication. Because compulsive distraction is the only way they've learned to escape from the painful feeling, these people need to learn mindfulness. There is an underlying tendency to create distraction in the mind. We are overwhelmed by the need for a narcotic once the habit has been established. Distraction may help temporarily, but in the long run people will lose their battle against pain. This battle, which is lived out through resistance, aversion, obsession, stress, and depression, is a road that goes nowhere except a worse place than before.

In summary, first comes the experience of pain, the basic unpleasant sensation, the primary first arrow, and temporary suffering when the problem is fixed.

Many respond with aversion, resistance, and resentment. Then people may use an avoidance strategy and complicate the distraction. People attempt to escape, but they end up in trouble with suffering and stress. People with chronic pain live a life of blocking, and its accompanying bad behaviors will eventually drown them. Blocking—using alcohol, cigarettes, drugs, shopping splurges, and experiencing withdrawal—are a few of the resistances in the attempt to escape the pain. People start spinning the wheel of avoidance, anxiety, and panic. Others drown in the process. Overwhelmed and exhausted, they give up, become depressed, stop exercising, and isolate themselves. An avoidance strategy may work for a while, but eventually people will wear out, become overwhelmed, and get worse.

A healthy response to pain is to become aware of the condition, not resist it, become distressed, or obsess about it. Holistic methods can stop the resistance, stop the blocking, and stop people's being overwhelmed by the symptoms. Mindfulness is a way to avoid blocking and drowning. People will become less responsive to the pain, pay less attention to it, and start leading a normal life. We need to move toward the acceptance of primary suffering and avoid the suffering from chronic pain problems. Remember the basic Buddhist philosophy, "Life is suffering." We will all face it sooner or later, and how we can enjoy life is totally dependent on how we handle the tough times that come to all of us at some time or another.

"Mindfulness is the key to breaking the habit of blocking and drowning in chronic pain." —*Living Well with Pain and Illness*, by Vidyamala Burch

The Nocebo in Action

The nocebo's effects are due to expectations of sickness. Years of this can result in mind-body illness and true, organic illness. Remember, illness is the perception of being unwell; although tests may reveal nothing, the symptoms are real. The nocebo effect can also cause real organic illness, physical changes in the body that can be demonstrated on tests. The word *nocebo* comes from the Latin word *nocere*, which means "I will harm." It is the opposite of the placebo effect, which means "I will heal."

The nocebo phenomenon is a little-recognized facet of culture and medicine that may be responsible for a substantial number of illnesses and diseases. It is dependent on how we speak to people. This could be a huge phenomenon in medicine, especially with the increasing amount of technology and laboratory tests available to providers. Overuse of this technology or interpretation of it can have great placebo effects and even more nocebo effects, resulting in unnecessary procedures and operations. The extent of the phenomenon is not yet known. I have personally asked 350 physicians and 300 others what the term nocebo means and I'm sad to say that no one knew. The concept of nocebo needs to be taught in medical school. In medicine we cause placebo and nocebo effects on patients all day long, changing people's perception of themselves continually. The nocebo effect was first described in 1960 and has been written about periodically in journals and books ever since. On the other hand, the placebo has been around for thousands of years. If people were to Google "placebo," they would get one million hits, compared to only a few hits on "nocebo."

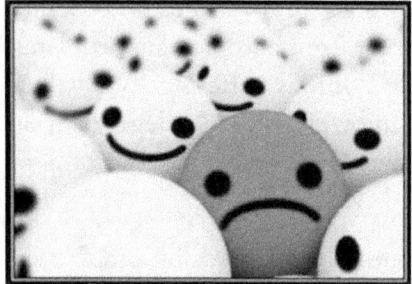

Some nocebo effects, such as a negative statement by a health care provider, may be transient. Others may be fatal. If a medical provider tells a cancer patient she is going to die in six months, odds are that she will. This is well documented in medical literature. But if people convert hopelessness to hopefulness, life span and cure rates increase, as Dr. Carl Simington and others have scientifically documented.

The nocebo effect is the cause of sickness by expectations of sickness or death, and by associated emotional states. Two forms of the nocebo effect have been recognized, the specific and generic forms. In the specific form, the patient expects a particular negative outcome and then it occurs. For example, my son, who is also a physician, had a patient who was told she was going to die within six months from a small malignant tumor in her brain. She went into panic mode and never recovered. She was dead in two days from stress-related cardiac arrhythmia. I describe her situation in more detail in a following chapter. Another example of the nocebo effect is a patient who expects to die on the operating table, and does. No one should operate on a patient who expects to die. Medical literature is full of stories on this phenomenon.

In the generic form, nocebo means that patients have a negative expectation. They are pessimistic, not hopeful, and their expectations are realized in the form of symptoms, mind-body illnesses, and occasionally death. Expectations cause changes to the neurotransmitters, hormones, and neuropeptides in the brain, to the autonomic nervous system and immune cells.

The physician can be a huge cause of the nocebo effect. How we speak to the patient and what the patient perceives can have devastating nocebo effects, or wonderful effects through the placebo. If the doctor is a good placebo, his words, appearance, and actions can lead to well-ness. The way that test results are discussed with the patient is critical. If the results of the CT, MRI, angiogram, or blood test are abnormal but appear unrelated to the patient's problem, the way a doctor conveys these results can induce an illness, disease, or even death. A healer can easily induce the nocebo effect, and how the patient thinks can affect the chemistry of his brain and body, resulting in illness and disease. The patient may undergo unnecessary procedures or operations because he was told that he has a serious back problem, or a vascular disease that is an incidental finding and has nothing to do with his chest pain or minor changes in his sinuses. Many times these findings with modern technology have nothing to do with the patient's problem. Thus we need to be very careful with our words. Many of these changes are due merely to aging and are unrelated to other health problems. I see this a great deal with angiograms and MRIs.

It has been my experience that medical providers receive no training in medical school about the effects of the mind on the body, or the effects of the body on the mind. Unfortunately, this is widely true in today's society. Recently, when I was at my forty-fifth medical school reunion, the dean asked if we had any questions. I had written a question on a piece of paper but it had been disregarded up to this point. So I took advantage of the situation, stood up, and addressed my question to the three brand-new doctors at the front. I asked, "What percentage of time do students spend learning about proper nutrition and wellness during their medical school careers?" The recent graduates said they had been taught this material a little bit in their sophomore year but that was all they could remember.

Seventy five percent of patients seen by a physician on any given day probably have a physical presentation of stress. Their test results are overdiagnosed as diseases that are actually related to stress and changes because of aging. This results in additional tests, injections, and possible surgeries. What those patients need is a coach, a wellness doctor, a doctor who cares, who is not trying to make money from test results—a placebo doctor. The effect of doctors with this nocebo attitudes is indescribable. Every day I see people wanting surgery when they don't need it, but another provider has told them that the operation may be necessary. If one's blood sugar is 500, for example, it clearly indicated diabetes, but many tests are not that clear. These unclear tests are used to convince people that something is wrong. Many tests can be abnormal but have nothing to do with the patient's problem. It should not be implanted into a patient's mind that there is something wrong. The nocebo phenomenon creates a culture of illness. We need to develop a culture of wellness. Eastern medicine is wellness-oriented. Western medicine is disease-orientated. When talking with a patient, every physician should include a discussion on wellness. Medical school courses should teach more about wellness. Physicians and schools may claim they have no time, but I don't believe that. I am seventy-three years old, practice neurosurgery full-time, perform surgery almost every day, read and write books every day, practice music, play tennis, give numerous lectures on wellness every week, run two yoga studios, and still have plenty of time to talk to my patients. We must make it a priority to talk to patients more. When medical schools admit students, they needn't choose geniuses; they need students who practice good health habits, have positive personalities, and possess the ability to care for the people who come to them for help. A caring, wellness-oriented, placebo doctor can cure seventy five percent of patients. We are creating carpenters and engineers of the human body, when the teaching of wellness and proper nutrition needs to be a huge part of medical school and of the board examinations. I'm sad to say that only two to three percent of our society are currently headed in that direction. Following this path would lead to better medical care, happier patients, and lower health care costs.

The Healer as an Agent of the Nocebo Effect

As people may now realize, how the healer communicates with people is very important. The patient's perception of illness or disease is easily affected by the words of the practitioner. In health care, the words used by the physician have a profound effect on the well-being of the patient. Words used by the physician can lead to healing, especially through the placebo effect. Unfortunately words can also lead to unnecessary medication, injections, and operations through the nocebo effect. Words can make people well and can make people believe, resulting in chemical changes in the brain and body that result in wellness. Or words can lead to a patient's becoming addicted to drugs or feeling anxious, fearful, or depressed.

One of my sons, who is a neurosurgeon, came to me one day and said, "Dad, I have a patient who I think represents what you are talking about." The patient was a thirty-five-year-old female with three children. She was divorced and was experiencing a lot of mental pressure. After having a seizure, she had an MRI scan that revealed a tumor.

It was not very large, but it was clearly malignant. She asked how long she had to live. He told her it would be about six months. No words of hope were used. She started screaming, and went into a state of panic that never stopped. The next day a biopsy was done, confirming the highly malignant tumor. Again she was told of the predicted outcome and no hopeful words were used, such as explaining that approximately ten percent of patients do very well for a number of years. The patient went into a state of hopelessness, and although the tumor was quite small, she was dead the next day. In essence, it was like the voodoo effect. The neuropeptides overwhelmed her body, blood pressure went up, and she went into heart failure. An autopsy revealed she had neurofibrillary degeneration. This was a very unfortunate situation, but it does prove the effects of how people think, possibly induced by a health provider who, in trying to be very honest, can induce the nocebo effect.

The language used can heal people or kill people. It can greatly change one's perception about what is really happening. The wrong words can produce despair and counteract the usefulness of whatever treatment is prescribed. Many times what the healer says is more important than the tests. Communication dominates the situation. The patient needs to know the reality of what is going on, but providers must give them some hope. No one can ever be one hundred percent certain about what is going to occur.

A number of years ago, I had a patient with a malignant brain tumor. When I gave him his diagnosis, he said, "I'm not going to die." He lived longer than any patient I ever had with that type of malignant brain tumor. I will never forget him. I took advantage of his way of thinking. I do everything to encourage anyone with the same diagnosis to live a very long time.

The physician's message may be clearly delivered and clearly understood, but the effect may run counter to the well-being of the patient. Not all patients are equally equipped to handle the truth and a healer must sense this. As exemplified in my son's case, confronting a patient at point-blank range with the reality of a life-threatening illness can have consequences the affect the patient's well-being. It could be said that the physician has no choice but to convey the facts flat out. Then he or she cannot be accused of failing to prepare the patient. But are the hard facts always necessary or useful? If at all possible, we should always try to convert hopelessness to hopefulness. It's part of healing. The wise physician will employ all the artistry in his or her power to potentiate and motivate the patient. The mind of the patient is extremely important in the healing process. Chemicals in the body are much different in an optimistic person compared to a pessimistic person. One attitude can lead to healing; the other can lead to death. The physician should try to avoid a situation in which a patient leaves the office

terrified, anxious, or depressed. Panic induced by a provider can be very harmful. If we treat only the illness, we've only treated half the problem. Panic can flood the heart with chemicals such as adrenaline, resulting in a heart attack. Many people with heart attacks never reach the hospital alive because of panic and the effect it has on the heart. Panic and stress through the entire endocrine system send the body into disarray.

The truth of patient's particular condition should not be denied or ignored, but we need to attach more importance to the manner and style of communication. Occasionally the patient is given the wrong medication or develops a complication from surgery, but I think our words cause an even greater incidence of damage. We induce the nocebo effect by what we say, by pessimism, or by overly interpreting modern technology. We turn the process of aging, as interpreted on MRIs and angiograms, into diseases. Many times these tests don't really explain what's going on, they merely adjust things that we see. Many psychological, iatrogenic, physician-induced illnesses are brought on by an emotional tailspin with physiological consequences, as result of an exchange with a healer.

Is it possible to communicate negative information in a way that is received by the patient as a challenge, rather than a death sentence? I believe we can communicate better without crippling the patient with negative news or overinterpreting highly technical studies. We should put our emphasis on the strategy of winning the battle. Physicians should ensure their patients that they are not going to let them die. Doctors can give a hug, propose a partnership, and outline a plan, put it in writing, and copy it for the patient. They can send patients to a wellness doctor who teaches mind-body techniques to improve healing. Doctors should provide patients with the best that science has to offer. There have been spontaneous cures and improvements with this type of treatment. For example, it has been proven and documented that cancer patients live twice as long by using mind-body techniques, and the rate of spontaneous cures increases. Most of the time we're not even talking about something as

serious as cancer, but an ordinary backache or headache where we induce negative thinking in the patient by overinterpreting diagnostic tests. This is the most common problem. The basic physician's purpose is not to destroy the hope that provides an essential environment for healing. The brain is the most powerful organ. It produces over three hundred neuropeptides and can heal or destroy. The rate of healing is always dependent on how one thinks. The mind plays a powerful part in health and illness. Most of these chemicals are activated by the patient's own attitudes and emotions. They are affected by the patient's self-confidence and his confidence in his physician, which can promote or destroy the will to live. Every serious illness is treatable and/or reversible, but the responsible physician wants to increase productive life and survival as much as possible. Most medical conditions are benign; they don't need heroics, they need a placebo, a wellness doctor who properly cares for her patient. My patients know that

I care about them. Patients want reassurance and they want people to listen. They want to know that their doctor cares whether they live or die. As providers, we must meet the emotional needs of the patient, and every patient is different. I personally think the crucial question when providers meet a patient is "What is going on in your life?" not, "Where does it hurt?"

All the CTs, MRIs, x-rays, medications and angiograms cannot substitute for the healer's role as the keeper of the keys to the body's own healing system. In reality, we all need a wellness doctor. Unfortunately, this subject is not taught in medical school very often. My hope is that everyone finds a wellness doctor. This wellness doctor lives within all of us. He or she just needs to be awakened!

History of the Nocebo

The relationship between the healer and the patient, what the healer says and what the patient asks, will determine whether that communication will have a positive or negative effect—a

placebo or a nocebo. It will help or it will harm. A negative statement may nullify the benefit of a doctor's treatments or even make an ill person feel worse. Combined, the personality and conviction of the healer, the hopeful attitude of the ill person, and a positive therapeutic relationship with the healer generate placebo effects. If the opposite occurs, negative statements, fearful statements, expectation of death, or the naming of diseases that are not actually present can have negative, or nocebo, effects. A doctor with a negative attitude toward a treatment for a patient may compromise the success of that patient's treatment. If your doctor does not spend time with you, or will not look you squarely in the eye, you may get a nocebo from the relationship. If he gives you a prescription and mentions a lot of potential side effects, he may be perfectly honest, but he destroys the placebo effect of the medication. I doubt you would receive the potential seventy percent placebo effect of the medication. If the nocebo effect is greater than the therapeutic gain and the natural history of the disease, the treatment will make you worse.

Dr. Walter Cannon was given the credit for research on acute stress. The acute stress response described the notion of voodoo death as a fatal power of the imagination working through unmitigated terror. These were the beliefs of aboriginal societies in Australia, New Zealand, Polynesia, and Africa. It is well known in Haiti that a powerful medicine man might cause death through fear. He points his finger at you, you believe it will kill you, and it does. Dr. Cannon believed that the voodoo death resulted from an overreaction of the sympathetic adrenaline autonomic nervous system's reaction to fear. This is an extreme example of the fight-or-flight phenomenon, for which Dr. Cannon is well known. Others have published medical papers suggesting that voodoo works through the parasympathetic nervous system and the autonomic nervous system's failure, the cause of death being cardiac arrhythmia. Modern scientists have localized the emotional component of fear to a part of the brain called the amygdala.

When Are Nocebo Attacks More Likely to Occur?

The more severe the symptoms, the worse the pain, and the more likely a placebo or nocebo will work. The roles of expectation and the emotional state of the person increase the likelihood of a placebo or nocebo effect. The greater the fearful anticipation that the shaman or witch doctor has the power to harm you, the more likely it will happen. A doctor or nurse can relieve symptoms through a positive attitude and a trustworthy relationship, or they can do harm through negative attitudes and lack of empathy. Worry, anxiety, stress, anger, and depression negatively influence health outcomes. Cynicism, suspicion, and a pessimistic expectation can generate negative outcomes such as illness and disease. A health care provider may be able to overcome the patient's pessimism with a positive attitude, or she can aggravate things with negative words. Making too much out of symptoms that may actually need very little treatment may lead to unnecessary surgery and reduce a patient's positive expectations. Self-scrutiny, as a result of our national plague of stress, can result in a variety of mind-body diseases. Certain illnesses such as irritable bowel syndrome, fibromyalgia, and atypical chest pain have no demonstrable basis. Medical students commonly develop negative symptoms when studying specific diseases and illnesses. About seventy five percent of patients with chest pain find stress is the cause. This is a nocebo effect from too much body scrutiny. Cardiac neurosis is a nocebo effect.

Negative medical tests can have a placebo effect, though failure to diagnose may also have a nocebo effect. If a patient is told that there is no accounting for his symptoms, he may begin to search for another doctor and look for a simple solution to make him well. Thus, some explanation must be given for the patient's symptoms. Generally, I use fairly benign terms like fibromyalgia or tension myositis. This means that nothing is seriously wrong and the patient has a treatable condition. I will treat this condition with education, stress-reduction techniques, and exercise, and have the patient look at my website and Dr. Rudy Kachmann's twenty prescriptions for stress reduction. Now the patient knows that something is wrong, but I have made her hopeful and reassured her that we are dealing with a benign condition. If I diagnose a patient with a mind-body disease like fibromyalgia, I spend a lot of time explaining it, giving the person things to read, reassuring him that the problem is not in his head, and I outline a treatment program. That's why I own two yoga studios that teach wellness. I have three hundred people in weight-management classes, taught by certified instructors, and I give the class a free lecture on wellness on a regular basis. I always recommend exercise. Taking a thirty-minute walk is as good as taking an antidepressant pill, in many cases. The modern patient wants facts—we worship at the altar of casualty and seek explanation, meaning, and recognition of our suffering. A physician should never doubt the patient's symptoms, even if she is skeptical when developing a plan for healing. Few things can make a patient angrier than hearing that her symptoms are in her head. Diagnosis demonstrates to the patient that his complaint is taken seriously, that it is a legitimate affliction, and that his suffering is recognized as genuine. The symptoms of mind-body illnesses and diseases are real. Diagnosis provides an understandable and satisfactory explanation for illness. Dismissive treatment of the symptoms can have nocebo effects, just as overstating causes of the symptoms can lead to surgery and persistent nocebo effects. An explanation gives some meaning to the illness, and its absence lessens the sense of well-being. Physicians need to avoid labeling people with an illness they don't have by over-reading their diagnostic studies.Let me give another example. My wife went to see an internist for the first time. She typed out a number of diagnoses and handed my wife the piece of paper which said, in bold, "**hypertension and hyperthyroidism**". Neither of these turned out to be correct, but they temporarily changed my wife's perception of herself.

I took her blood pressure the next morning. It was 100 over 70, and her thyroid test was normal. She was given a prescription for hypertension. I told her not to take it until we got a few readings. Perception is everything; the words we use are everything.

This diagnosis of diseases is a byproduct of specialization. We now have organ doctors who focus their knowledge on one organ, not the whole body. The same medical symptoms can produce a variety of diagnoses, depending on which specialists people see. Whereas I may tell people they have a mind-body disease, one specialist may tell them they have a bowel disease, and another may say the gallbladder is causing problems and needs to be removed. A surgeon would want to do an exploratory operation and would take the gallbladder out. Very few doctors consider the whole body or practice holistic medicine. A holistic doctor takes a long medical history, finds out what's going on in the patient's life, allows patients to participate in their own care, provides a lot of alternatives, and doesn't diagnose when there's very little evidence for the condition. Just because you have gallbladder stones, kidney stones, or lumbar degenerative disc disease doesn't mean that this is the cause of your back pain. It needs to be proven. You should see a holistic doctor. Few doctors are equipped to take care of the patient's fundamental psychological problems, as very little is taught about this in medical school. Most doctors are not trained in proper nutrition. A specialist is a specialist, each with a narrow view of a single organ. Once a test of that organ is exhausted, the patient moves on, disappointed in his quest to understand the meaning of various symptoms.

What Is the Placebo?

I believe that most people perceive the placebo as a medication that has no inherent value, but when it is perceived as valuable, it can have an effect. In fact, a placebo can come in many forms, such as a person, a doctor, or a health care provider. Because patients value the provider's opinion, she has the ability to heal people. As a matter of fact, a placebo can also be a procedure, test, injection, or an operation. A great deal of the effectiveness of a placebo is due to the patient's perception. For example, my patients have commented many times that I'm the best-dressed man in town. I've always liked nice ties, foreign shoes, and fancy suits. Why? They make me feel good and, in turn, make my patients feel confident in my ability to help them. I'm one hundred percent convinced that my style of dress has a placebo effect on my patients. Their attitude changes immediately. They think I'm successful and thus they believe that I can heal them. Perception is extremely important.

Let me give another example of a person being healed by a procedure that had no inherent value. I was treating a very successful president of a company who had severe sciatic nerve pain that should have been the result of a ruptured disc. I tried various types of nonsurgical treatment to heal him, including medication, physical therapy, a chiropractor, hot tubs, and exercise. None of the nonsurgical therapies worked. The patient's x-rays and MRI were completely normal. I told him that there was no clear-cut evidence of a ruptured disc. He told me that if I didn't do something he would have to close his small factory and put thirty people out of work. Sometimes a ruptured disc can be hidden and people can find it during surgery, in spite of a normal x-ray. So I operated on him and found absolutely nothing. At that point I had to think as a healer. Instead of telling him that I didn't find anything, I told him that I took the pressure off the nerve and removed some arthritis. I was stretching a point, but he was back at work in two days. The operation had a placebo effect, since I found nothing during surgery.

The placebo effect goes beyond the physical realm. I view it as the belief of the patient that changes the chemistry of his brain; causes the secretion of hormones, neurotransmitters, and neuropeptides; and results in the patient getting well again.

The history of medicine before the 1900s reveals the history of the placebo effect, according to Dr. William Osler, a famous physician. The word placebo comes from the Latin word *placere,* which means "I will please." Originally it was a medication prescribed to satisfy the patient, not because the doctor thought it would do any real good. Procedures involving bloodletting, leeches, snakes, frogs, and all sorts of creatures were also used for their placebo effect. These placebos were inert substances given as a medication. They were an inactive substance given to satisfy an increased demand for medication. Many times it worked, but sometimes it caused harm, as with bloodletting. George Washington, the first president of the United States of America, died from bloodletting. Believe it or not, though, sometimes it worked. A century ago Dr. Osler said, "One should treat as many patients as possible with the new drug while it still has the power to heal." He was clearly referring to the placebo effect of medication that has no inherent value. In other words, there is no scientific proof that a placebo works. It is only the belief of the patient that makes it work, especially the way it is presented by the health care provider.

Any therapy, including injections, surgery, diet, natural medicine, devices, and procedures, can produce the placebo effect. Placebos have been employed since the beginning of medicine and I believe they should be part of everyday practice. Over the years, fifty percent to seventy five percent of the patients I've seen needed wellness teaching and could have benefited from the placebo, if it were presented by a healer who cared about the patient. This would remove the risk of taking a lot of medication and enduring procedures. We need a lot of wellness medical practitioners to take advantage of the placebo effect, and not be a nocebo to their patient. The ancient Chinese had approximately 2,500 medications in their formularies. They healed a lot of patients, but mostly through inert medications without a lot of side effects. Prior to World War II, the deliberate use of inert medications was part of everyday medicine.

History of the Mysterious Placebo

The placebo effect has been used for centuries. The prescription is a certificate for assured recovery and patients expect it. The trick is to give the patient only a few of the least risky kind of pill you can find. I believe that the doctor should use a true placebo pill. She should try to find some type of safe medication from a health food store. I keep a list in my office and refer to it when I'm treating a fairly benign pain problem and the patient's perception seems out of sync with the reality of the situation. I use chemicals that have only mild to moderate effect, but because of the patient's high expectations, they usually work. I help the patient without taking a major risk or getting them addicted to narcotics. I think every healer needs a few medications to use when he sees the right situation to help the patient get better without harming them or leading to addiction.

Taking advantage of the placebo effect is completely ethical. It is simply a tool to help the patient, not fool them. The body knows how to get well and remembers wellness. Dr. Herbert Benson likes to call the placebo effect "remembered wellness." I think he is right. Norman Cousins said, "Most people seem to feel their complaints are not taken seriously unless they are in possession of a little slip of paper with indecipherable magic markings." The prescription is the doctor's IOU of good health, but drugs are not always necessary. Belief in recovery is always necessary, yet a prominent message from the medical community is that the practice of medicine must be based on scientific proof and double-blind studies or evidence-based medicine. What they have done is essentially cut the brain out of the human body, as René Descartes did three hundred years ago. They have not gotten over this practice. The medical community seems to have forgotten the effects of the human mind and the patient's perception of his or her medical problem.

The success of healers throughout the ages must be evaluated in regards to the capacity for self-healing that exists in all living beings. The mechanisms of spontaneous recovery from physical and mental disease are not always completely understood. We do not know everything the neurotransmitters, hormones, and neuropeptides produced by the brain and body can do to us. In her famous book *Molecules of Emotion*, Candace Pert discusses this subject in detail. How we think has a tremendous effect on our well-being. Pert discusses how our brain speaks to our body through neurotransmitters, hormones, and neuropeptides, and our body speaks to our brain through the same chemicals. The monocytes of the blood make all the same neurotransmitters, hormones, and neuropeptides—brain to body, body to brain.

The mental attitude of a patient has a lot to do with the course of their disease. How we think can affect our immunity. Stress can cause cancer. But in some cases, positive thinking can cure cancer. A more hopeful patient will do far better than a pessimistic patient, so how we speak to a patient is extremely important. We can induce a placebo or a nocebo effect. A healer who does not know how to communicate with the patient has no placebo effect; they should probably be a radiologist or a pathologist, or not go into medicine in the first place. Medical school admissions committees need to know the personalities of the students they admit to medical school. They don't need geniuses; they need students who like people and who are good communicators and motivators. That's what makes a hero.

The secretion of hormones, neurotransmitters, and neuropeptides positively or negatively affects emotional states. Because stress can destroy the human body, a good doctor-patient relationship is very important. There needs to be a partnership between the physician and patient. The only way to improve the health care system is through the partnership of wellness. The patient must assume some responsibility for his or her own well-being, but the healer must teach the patient the way. After all, the word *physician* means "teacher."

Modern medicine will become even more scientific when physicians and their patients have learned to manage the forces of the body and the mind. Medicine is very scientific, but it needs to make great strides in conjunction with the chemicals in the human mind.

A placebo pill given by a doctor appears to be more powerful than one given by a nurse or clerk. A placebo injection is more powerful than a placebo pill. A large pill is more effective than a small pill, and a very small pill is better than a regular-sized pill. The color and size of pills also affect the placebo response. Capsules are more effective than tablets. Yellow pills are for depression and green ones are for anxiety. Placebo is believed to be blocked by the narcotic antagonist naloxone, proving the placebo effect of medication. Placebo can be caused by one's own endorphins.

Over the centuries nearly anything people could imagine has been tried as a placebo. Some of these substances were fads and frauds. That is why today a placebo medication would need to be given by an experienced physician who knows scientific medicine, applies it appropriately, and is not trying to use it to make a living. Physicians must exercise good judgment by not substituting a placebo for a scientifically proven medication, but using a placebo properly really works.

I find that the nocebo effect doctors are having on their patients through modern medical technology, chemistry, and procedures is doing a great deal of harm. I'm not worried about the placebo effect, I'm merely pointing out how to take advantage its benefits. Many times we can get patients well again without a lot of heroics. On the other hand, negative talk can surely make them sicker and lead to unnecessary procedures. The placebo is the good twin and the nocebo is the evil twin.

How Do Placebos and Nocebos Work?

Hormones, neurotransmitters, and neuropeptides are secreted by the brain, as are monocytes in the blood. They are responsible mechanisms connected with the circuits in the cerebral cortex. A variety of modes of action such as suggestion, conditioning, and stimuli from all our senses become possible. The desired response may be conditioned through training, whether in an animal or a human. Biofeedback is an example of that. The doctor may be the biggest placebo or nocebo. The degree to which he or she is able to induce the placebo or nocebo has a tremendous effect on the situation. The greater the patient's need for help, the more likely it will result in a positive or negative response, and that response may be elicited without the patient's conscious awareness. The meaningful experience, which is very important, can, through cortical mechanisms, induce widespread bodily changes and heal or harm the patient. The administration of medication has meaning for the patient, and the effect varies from person to person because we all think differently. Anyone can introduce a new drug or pill and it may work for a long time, but it may be difficult to remove or destroy an old remedy, even after it has stopped working. For example, bloodletting seemed to stay around for centuries despite its adverse effects.

The End Point

Life has a beginning and an end. Believe it or not, so do most pain problems. It actually depends a great deal on you and your provider. If addictive pain medication is not stopped in time you will become tolerant of it, develop a dependency on it, and eventually become addicted to it. Pain centers will claim that the likelihood of the chronic usage of narcotics leading to addiction is extremely low, but I completely disagree. Why do we have people dying all around us from physician-prescribed drugs? We did not have this before the fifth vital sign was established. Now they have to measure the fifth vital sign—pain in the hospital—and the merry-go-round begins. We no longer decide if the medication is needed; instead the nurse says, "What's your level of your pain, 0 to 10?" and off we go. Diagnosis is irrelevant. How stupid can you get?

If we're going to use the fifth vital sign, let's establish the sixth vital sign. The sixth vital sign should be the plan for when to stop the medication. We need to know the endpoint at the beginning or the process will continue forever. Now the patient leaves the hospital with addictive medication, sees another doctor, and the band plays on. That is what is establishing the huge population of habituated and addicted people—no endpoint was established at the start of treatment. There was no plan in place. It is not the undertreatment of pain that is causing this epidemic. Neuropathic pain, anatomically based pain, and pain based on nerve damage are only a small part of the nation's pain problems. Pain may be occasionally undertreated in the beginning, but it has been scientifically proven that narcotics help only about thirty percent of the people, thirty percent of the time—the "30/30 rule".

In the majority of cases, pain problems are never aggressively treated with mind-body techniques that essentially have no side effects and are very effective in majority of patients. I noticed in the latest pain book I read that mind-body techniques were at the back of the book, when they should have been at the front of the book. No one dies from mind-body techniques, and hardly anyone advocating these techniques is ripping the system off—there's not much money in wellness studios; most barely breakeven. They just help people with relatively safe techniques. Undoubtedly some patients are occasionally overtreated with, for example, chiropractic visits. But that's a lot better than injections, narcotics, or surgeries. We may not know the endpoint but we should have a plan from the beginning. People should not be permitted to come to the emergency room for a shot for nonneuropathic chronic pain. The majority the time the hospital starts running diagnostic tests test, CTs, and MRIs to protect themselves legally and to make some money. Most of the time it just results in a three-page report producing a nocebo on the patient, who reads the report, carries it home, and obsesses about it, making things worse, all the while filling the prescription for narcotics that were not needed in the first place, and the addictive process begins or continues.

For acute pain, narcotic prescriptions should be used for a month or less. For chronic pain there should be a plan. The plan should not be sending people to any old pain center. Don't start with injections and end up with narcotics; I see this tragedy a great deal of the time. I see it almost every day. Certainly there are some exceptions, but a holistic pain center is difficult to find. Just check pain centers' websites—you don't see much advertising for a holistic approach. It's all about procedures and medications. How many have a psychologist on their staff? Psychologists need to be part of the team. How many physical therapists do they have? How many massage people do they have? There's no money in these treatments, so they are not available. The fact that these treatments are not as profitable does not mean pain centers have the right to treat people with the moneymaking stuff without a holistic approach to treatment.

I see many patients who started with an acute pain problem and were given strong medication that was never stopped and now they have a second disease, "chronic pain," established by their previous medication because it caused the development of neural circuits in the brain which are now causing real pain. The pain center may say providers are undertreating pain, but people will never get off narcotics unless doctors help them and treat them in a more holistic manner.

When narcotics are given for a few weeks, new receptor sites develop within the brain, new neural circuits develop, and in the absence of the medicine the patient develops withdrawal symptoms. Then he makes a phone call to his doctor or goes to the emergency room seeking a refill and the primacy of the condition is established.

Many of these patients will become anxious or depressed, and some even commit suicide. Just read the paper and you will see this day after day. Look at all the famous people who died from this process.

When I walk down the hall of a pain center close to me in the hospital, the waiting room is so full people are hanging out in the hallway. I see them all in the elevator and they all look alike. Most are young, have tattoos, smell like smoke, and look pale and glassy-eyed. This goes on day after day. These are the addicts as established by the pain doctor, or before he ever saw them. The Rolodex keeps on rolling. A doctor who works across the hall has completely confirmed my impression. I feel sorry for the patients; I suspect many of their lives are ruined. How many of them do you think have an endpoint to the treatment plan? I would be surprised to find even one. Dumping pain patients into the system is ridiculous. What's the point? The first prescription should be accompanied with a plan, an endpoint, the sixth vital sign. Meanwhile, a lot of people are making a lot of money prescribing narcotics—emergency room staff ordering tests that cost thousands, some for good reason but many leading to nothing except overtreatment; lawyers filing lawsuits over pain from accidents that are difficult to prove; patients applying for disability because of chronic pain of unclear etiology; the pharmaceutical industry making a fortune; and unnecessary procedures making people a lot of money. Everyone given a narcotic prescription should have an endpoint.

The Heart of Addiction: The Addictive Thought System

Fear is the root of addictive behavior. Egos make it up; the core of addictive behavior is fear. There are four fundamental parts to the addictive system. They are fear, living in the past or the future, judgment, and belief in scarcity.

Fear

According to Dr. Lee Jampolsky, there are four fundamental parts of the addictive thought system. Dr. Jampolsky has never seen addictive behavior without fear. That is a bold statement but one that makes a lot of sense. Fear is the fuel that the addictive thought system runs on. Instead of inviting love we become hosts to guilt. Guilt causes us to have many faulty and negative beliefs about ourselves.

Living in the Past or Future

In the addictive thought process system we stockpile ammunition used to condemn others and ourselves. We manufacture "a guilt bomb." Resentment turns into sandbags on our back. We spend fifty percent over our time worrying about the future; we spend two hundred thoughts a day about what we're going to eat. That's found in the medical literature.

Judgment

While judging, you cannot love. While you love, you cannot judge. Life is not an experiment. We are taught judgment and analysis of the hallmarks of knowledge and wisdom. Whenever they make a negative judgment you are making a choice to experience conflict rather than peace. Many of us have a problem with the relentless grip of judgment squeezing the joy and love out of our relationships. This results in a lot of guilt, the hallmark of addictive behavior. You must learn to love yourself. When you forgive yourself and remember who you are, you will bless everyone and everything you see. You cannot judge and have peace of mind at the same time. When you extend love, you receive love. In an addictive thought system, the day starts with condemnation and judgment. But with practice you can just as easily choose to fill your mind with love.

Scarcity

Much of our emotional pain comes from thinking that we are lacking. We search for a sense of wholeness. We need something to fill the void. We need self-love and self-acceptance. Whenever people are holding onto the past or worrying about the future, they are looking nowhere, seeing things that are not there.

In summary, I am concerned that the forty percent of the people with chronic pain are improperly treated with narcotics instead of cognitive training, exercise, and mind-body techniques, which will be discussed in detail in another chapter, as well as occasional nonnarcotic medications. In these forty percent of the people who have metabolic Pain (centralized brain pain) symptoms, you find no medical condition, and they are prone to become addicted to narcotics. They are the victims of the pain center. They receive many injections, then addictive drugs, which they justify to themselves based on the nocebo of providers and their diagnostic tests which, though not related to the patient's symptoms, have created a hugely profitable industry.

Pain Is not a Diagnosis

I always say that the gold standard of pain treatment is not the word of the patient. It is easy to estimate our own pain inaccurately, and pain perception differs from person to person, among the sexes, among the races, and among cultures. So to use the word of the patient, the number of the scale of 0 to 10, as a good standard of treatment makes no sense. We give narcotics to people with an undiagnosed pain problem and sixty to seventy percent of the time it habituates and addicts them, as I very commonly see.

I recommend that we use diagnosis with a clear cause as the focus of treatment. You have to know what you are dealing with. Certainly using pain medication like a narcotic for a week or two, maybe even a month, is occasionally necessary while tests are being run to determine the source of the pain. But when we've reached an endpoint, the medication needs to be stopped to avoid addiction, habituation, or sensitization of the body causing the need for stronger medicines.

Recently I read a book called *The Culture of Pain*, by David B. Morris. In it he states, "We should use pain as a diagnosis." He thinks that should be the new national standard. To me, that's exactly what the pain centers have been doing and they're addicting my whole city. They are addicting the whole country. The pain industry has taken over. Anyone can say they have pain. Clearly the whole country needs more dopamine, but we should not be getting it from narcotics. We should be getting it from laughter, exercise, and numerous other holistic ways of getting well again. We are creating a "pain" society because of a lack of serotonin and dopamine. It is horrible to say to a patient, "My diagnosis is pain." I say we need to have more than a diagnosis, a cause of pain. I'm talking about a reason for one's pain. Pain is a symptom, a sensation, a perception, and should not be used as a diagnosis which could lead and has led to what I witnessed at the pain centers. I walked through one the other night and found the addicts lying on the floor in the hallway waiting to get the magic prescription from a place where the doctor talked to them for thirty seconds and created these addicts. This is occurring across the whole country. Remember, the biggest cause of drug addiction in this nation is physician prescriptions. If you don't think so, visit a pain center and sit among the people. Certainly there are a few exceptions, but read the newspapers and you will find discover the number of deaths related to the diagnosis of pain.

The Future of Chronic Pain

You cannot deny that chronic pain is a perception, a sensation, and an emotion. Pain is in the mind and the body. We have attached the brain and body to chronic pain.

There has been a debate going on between the central (brain) and peripheral (spinal cord) theories of the causation of chronic pain. One is more brain oriented and the other more spinal cord oriented. Let's face it, there is not much money in the brain aspect of pain, and I suspect that that is having an influence. We don't do frontal lobotomies anymore. Yet we perform many spinal procedures at the pain centers, sometimes a hundred a day. I have seen it. Pain centers spend the rest of the day addicting people to narcotics to ensure repeat business.

Conditions that frequently accompany chronic pain include divorce, rape, abuse, incest, depression, grief, alcoholism, suicide, drug addiction, unemployment, job loss, bankruptcy, and toxic families. Chronic pain patients also have generally a complex psychological history before and after the chronic pain begins.

The future of chronic pain will involve both physical and psychological aspects. It cannot be solved completely by injection or a procedure. The placebo effect of doing something certainly can be great, but the effect lasts only a month or two.

Pain is affected by cognitive influences. It has different meanings to different people, different cultures, different races, and different sexes. Every single person perceives chronic pain differently. Remember, the words I recommend when first seeing a patient are not "where do you hurt," they are "what's going on in your life?" The approach needs to be a mind, body, and spirit approach, not just throwing narcotics, pain stimulators, or all sorts of other invasive procedures at the problem. If the pain is mainly "central," what good is it to do something to the spinal cord? That's why we see poor results. Chronic pain is a psycho-physiological reaction. Pain is a symbolic event of what's going on in a person's life. It overlaps with the personal and cultural need to have a meaningful life. Developing meaning helps us but it may not cure the condition. Pain is arrow one, arrow two, or both. The spinal injection may help for a few days, but most of time it's just a placebo event.

What does the immediate future hold for chronic pain? Pain clinics are not the answer because they're all different; some are greedy, and the staff and methods of treatment differ greatly from center to center. Very few offer low-risk, low-cost approaches. The risk of quackery cannot be dismissed since pain is a big moneymaker, and many insurance companies now pay for six months of treatment.

The origin of chronic pain often is murky and that really is a big problem. Once pain has been in the brain for six months, it is not the same as it was in the beginning. What about what I call metabolic Pain (centralized brain pain), pain without clear cause. Books by authors like Dr. Wilson, Dr. Thurston, Dr. Dillard, Dr. Blakely don't even mention those people we see almost daily that have been "noceboed" by their health care provider into thinking there's something wrong within the body that explains the pain and provides the excuse for them to do something, when in reality it has nothing to do with their problem.

It may very well turn out that relief will only arrive when we take charge of it ourselves. We need to think, develop a plan, and try listing methods in the beginning and at the end for a better outcome. Narcotics are not the answer. We need to take personal responsibility for the meaning of the pain. We must learn to think in spite of pain. We must work inside of every emotion, feeling, and perception. Education may be the key. That is why I have CDs, DVDs, lectures, and books available. The informed patient is most likely to change; I must admit, it is extremely difficult to change the habituated or addicted patient who may have overwhelming craving or even change his behavior to get the medication he wants.

The definition of chronic pain needs to change, and I think it will take a war because of the money in it. The federal laws governing narcotic prescriptions should be changed; that is probably the only thing that could change provider activity, which is at this moment the largest cause of drug addiction and drug-related deaths across the nation.

The Drug from Hell: OxyContin

Overdosing on OxyContin, abused or not abused, in combination with antidepressants and/or tranquilizers, leads to the coroner's office on a daily basis in the US. Of course, when taken as recommended by Purdue by cancer patients or people with true neuropathic pain, OxyContin can give very gratifying pain relief. Nonetheless, it contributes to fifteen thousand annual opiate deaths and huge numbers of legal addicts, all through providers who write prescriptions for opiate and opioid medications. Is this a war? I would certainly say it is, and it's getting worse by the months and years.

In the 1990s, oxycodone, a synthetic opioid, was developed. Derived from opiates (morphine), it produced products like Percocet, Percodan, Tylox, and eventually OxyContin, this last being a great deal stronger and more dangerous. It seemed like a perfect solution—great pain relief with a low habituation and addiction rate. But this idea was dead wrong. It was heavily advertised by Purdue Pharma. Providers started prescribing it like it was candy. I completely remember the beautiful saleslady who spoke to me a number of times. I must admit I never fell for the product, although I certainly gave the saleslady a second look. Oxycodone-based drugs like Percocet, Percodan, Tylox, and OxyContin were introduced in the mid-1990s by Purdue Pharma. OxyContin tablets contain substantially larger doses of oxycodone. Percocet, Percodan, and Tylox contain about 5 mg of oxycodone, versus 100–150 mg in OxyContin. Unfortunately, OxyContin was heavily marketed even for plain old backaches besides the more serious problems like cancer or broken bones. Indeed, OxyContin seemed like a miracle drug, but tolerance, habituation, and addiction soon followed.

It costs about $400 for a month's supply for a prescription of OxyContin, which is often covered by insurance. That's about fifty cents for a pill that could be resold for $40 to $80 a pill. A prescription for a hundred pills, sold on the street as it is commonly done, is worth $4000 to $8000. You can see the point. Patients speak about this a great deal in pain center waiting rooms and in the government-paid taxicabs that take them home. Significant numbers of physicians also saw the potential to make some money through narcotic prescriptions. Some of them are in jail today and there are more to come. I know that because I've spoken to a federal DEA agent, and he said they watch pain centers on a regular basis. Some of these unscrupulous doctors could even be put in jail for a lifetime, and justifiably so, because they gave prescriptions inappropriately, resulting in many deaths. I've visited the coroner's office in various counties on more than one occasion. Many of these habitually addicted patients are selling their pills on the street because they are very poor and frankly need money to pay the rent. They have told me so. Addiction leads to poverty, and it is especially upsetting when the process was started by a physician. Sometimes the first prescription, an unnecessary narcotic like Vicodin, can set addiction in motion. Pain centers are especially good at this; I see it on a regular basis. If you don't believe it, just read my patient's stories in their own words in this book.

OxyContin, taken correctly twice daily, can give great pain relief. The requirement, though, is that you actually have a neuropathic pain problem or pain caused by nerve damage or cancer—not some minor change on an x-ray; not chronic pain from depression, anxiety, hopelessness, and anger. Patients often can't tell the difference, so they are dependent on the provider to be an honest individual. Conservative modalities should be offered on a regular basis and should be listed on pain centers' websites. The prescription or injection should not be the first choice for most cases. But we don't see a lot of that. The profit motive is at work.

OxyContin is released slowly over a twelve-hour period. It can help the patient with cancer or with clear-cut nerve damage. Then it is a wonder drug, but that is not the reason it is given most of the time. Most the time it's given to patients with metabolic Pain (centralized brain pain), pain of unclear etiology, much of it due to anxiety, fear, anger, and hopelessness. In these troubled economic times it's almost understandable. OxyContin causes an immediate high, which makes people feel relaxed and numb. Who couldn't use a dose of that? But if the award is habituation and addiction, including death sometimes, it certainly is not worth it. Let's find other ways to relieve our pain, including exercise, music, laughter, love, or family. Addicts steal from the family and think nothing about it; that's the addictive process. When OxyContin is used in ways not intended by the provider, like when patients cut their pills in half, it is highly addictive. Yet OxyContin is handed out readily by many pain centers. Just read my patients' stories—and I know of many more.

Altering OxyContin to increase its effect quickly has become an epidemic. One out of twenty teenagers is doing it—how horrible. OxyContin was quickly called "hillbilly heroin" and paid for by insurance companies, Medicaid, and Medicare. Incidentally, Medicaid has no deductible for a physician's visit. If people are really sick this lack of deductible is a wonderful thing, but if they are ripping off the system it can cause the taxpayer a lot of headaches. I've had many family doctors complain to me about this. With no deductible, patients are running to the doctor for just about anything. The government even pays for the taxi service to take them to the provider, a privilege the taxpayer does not enjoy. Taxpayers are foolish to put up with it, and many don't know about it. I'm blowing the whistle on that fraud! In many states methadone clinics treat more OxyContin patients than heroin addicts. Compared to OxyContin, heroin costs less, but insurance doesn't pay for it. On the street, however, OxyContin is the cheaper drug. When the scripts run out, heroin comes up to bat. The withdrawal symptoms of OxyContin are severe headaches or migraines, severe sweating, diarrhea, and chest pain, and sometimes the heart stops and people don't wake up. OxyContin is also known as "Oxy," "OC," or even "killer" or "hillbilly heroin." One in twenty high school students admits to taking "oxy," and use has increased forty percent in these students. OxyContin has been a great source of drug trading among teenagers. Many steal from it from their relatives, or steal money from their families to pay for it. People buy it at a pharmacy for fifty cents and then sell it for $40 to $80 a pill. No wonder teenagers are driving better-looking cars.

A person might ask, "Do the benefits of OxyContin outrank the complications?" Let's face it, it's no contest. We have many other medications that could treat the pain of even cancer. Let's keep OxyContin for cancer; we don't need it for the rest. Pain generally does not kill you, but drug addiction can, along with the other tranquilizers and relaxers. Let the cancer specialists handle prescriptions, and take OxyContin away from the providers who are abusing it. I trust the cancer doctors but not the pain center doctors, not most of them. There is no secondary gain for the cancer physician. If sticking needles in patients is so great for pain, how come the cancer doctors are not doing it? Generally the pain pumps help the cancer patients, and I do recommend it for them. But overall, the "miracle drug" we thought would solve the chronic pain dilemma turned into a nightmare for many people. Some died, and a significant number are now living in poverty and permanent addiction. Many of them live in the street. Purdue Pharma mailed out fourteen thousand videos called "I Got My Life Back," in which doctors and nurses claim OxyContin is a miracle drug. We need another follow-up video called "Let's Have a Second Look at OxyContin." There was $1.5 billion in sales of OxyContin 2005, 1.5 million prescriptions alone.

OxyContin especially should never be given to people with a history of drug abuse. All patients should be tested for drug abuse before doctors even consider writing such a prescription, and then it should be given only for clear-cut neuropathic pain or cancer. If you read the pages written by my patient, it will surely will make you cry or get mad. I've done both. What is even more shameful is that we doctors are supposed to be healers and we're taking normal people and making addicts out of them. Then the government turns around and pays for it all through Medicaid and Medicare. If this is corrected nationally we could probably save $1 billion a year when you add up the total cost of medication, hospitalization, nursing home care, divorce, job loss, and accidents. I recently saw a patient who was a quadriplegic who will never walk again, and it's completely related to the medication he received at a pain center. He didn't die, but that would be even more expensive. It will probably cost the government millions if he lives about ten years. Just look at the human suffering to the patient and his family, all of which was preventable if the patient and provider had done the right things. Somebody needs to stand up to bat. Please join me!

Methadone: Darling of the Pain Management Community

Methadone clinics are abounding all over the country. They have a bad reputation, according to a federal agent I spoke to, as well as to patients and providers. Methadone is used supposedly as a step-down drug from heroin and opiates. The craving is not as high and the withdrawal symptoms are not as severe, but it still affects the narcotic circuitry of the brain. The particular problem with that is that it takes a long time for methadone to leave the blood and it has a prolonged metabolic half-life. It blocks the NMDA receptors. This is why there has been a resurgence of methadone use for the treatment of chronic pain. Remember, narcotics build an increased number of receptors in the brain, and these hungry receptors want to be fed or you get withdrawal symptoms. This is because you develop tolerance, and the same dose no longer gives you a high or returns you to normal feeling. In 2007, four million prescriptions were written in this country. This resulted in many deaths and overdoses as well as many disabled people. Many were left with major complications resulting in job loss and life in a nursing home. The number of overdose deaths resulting from opiates exceeded deaths from car accidents. Some people just don't wake up because of methadone's long half-life. Methadone plays a disproportionate role in such deaths. Dr. Joan Christy says, "The intention to better manage chronic pain with methadone and other agents has led to what has been described as a rising tide of deaths."

Methadone also affects the electrical conduction system of the heart. An expert panel has established actual standards with five recommendations for cardiac monitoring. They highly recommend checking the blood level frequently. The point is that sudden cardiac death can occur even when you keep these medications below the recommended blood level. Methadone especially affects the cardiac electrical conduction system when it interacts with tranquilizers, antidepressants, and other neuroleptic agents. It stays in the blood from five to eighty-nine hours, a potentially dangerous situation. Blood levels can build up and should be checked frequently. Interaction with other drugs, especially opiates, can be life threatening and cause cardiac and respiratory complications or even death. Alcohol and benzodiazepines particularly react to methadone in the blood. The point is that prevention should be the mainstay of treatment.

The Bottom Line: $$$ - Nocebo-Placebo Procedure

The nocebo plays a huge part in medicine. We nocebo (speak about the negative) all day long just by what we say, and when we use the CT scans, MRI scans, angiograms, x-rays, and just plain old words to convince people that their symptoms are related to the results of those tests. Sometimes that is the case, and a lot of the time it may not be intentional. The degenerative disease can be the cause of their pain problem, or it could be the slightly abnormal vascular angiogram that is the cause of their symptoms, thus promoting a lot of procedures that may or not be necessary. The procedure may be done because of the nocebo. The patient believes the procedure will work, and it does for a period of time. The nocebo, the reason given by the provider, leads to the procedure; the patient believes in its usefulness through the placebo effect and thus gets better for a period of time. I see it all the time—the doctor in these cases is really a great engineer or technician, but not an honest one, and the placebo keeps them in business. After a few months the patient's pain is back, along with a new set of symptoms, and the merry-go-round of mind-body illnesses starts all over again. That's where the money is. There is not much money in holistic teaching. I know, because I do it every day. That's just fine because I'm doing my job as a physician, remembering that physician means "teacher." I give multiple lectures to my patients every day, and we listen to CDs, watch DVDs, and read books. Believe me, there's no money in the latter, just a lot of bills, but it sure makes me feel good. Many patients feel better for a period of time after they have a procedure done because they believe it will work. I see it all the time. Two to three months later the patient is walking up and down the mind-body index and seeing another doctor, many times in a different specialty, and the nocebo and placebo start over again.

Providers must understand mind-body medicine, holistic medicine, but none of this is taught in medical school. I had a chiropractic student around for a few days last week and I could not believe it, he knew nothing of mind-body medicine, either. He knew basic science very well but didn't seem to realize the brain is attached to the body. I'd think it would be natural for a chiropractic student to understand this, but it is not. I'm happy to say that I do know quite a few chiropractors who indeed practice mind-body medicine. They frequently invite me to give lectures to their associations, and I appreciate that.

The human body and mind can give us false signals. At least seventy percent of the time chronic pain is a reflection of anxiety, stress, fear, depression, and the bumps and bruises of life! It's just plainly a fraud. Chronic pain doesn't kill anybody and should not be the plague that it is to many people. Nocebo-placebo proceduralists are extremely common and you must beware of them. They may be excellent in their technique and get away with a lot of the stuff because they're good at it, but the necessity of these techniques is another matter altogether.

Rudy Kachmann's Holistic Pain Clinic

It's one thing to criticize the majority of today's pain clinics, but another to recommend a better one. The reason for starting a holistic pain clinic is to get away from all these procedures and addictive medications and make the patient well, with less risk and cost. I don't think it would be easy to open a freestanding holistic pain clinic. I doubt a surgical group would ever do such a thing. I doubt hospitals would support it financially. I have one in a hospital, but I'm the owner of it. Hospitals could make money from these clinics, but they get paid for procedures, that's where the real money is. The majority of patients with severe chronic pain have no money. Many are addicts, and a number of them are physically or psychologically disabled.

My mind-body institute is working fairly well because I'm in a hospital and its main focus is wellness, not just pain. I'm developing a holistic pain clinic within it. I already have available a lot of the wellness modalities, like massage, yoga, tai chi, mindfulness, personal training, weight reduction, and zumba. The director of a pain clinic must have a thorough underlying understanding of wellness and pain, and money cannot be the primary goal. The pain centers today that do a lot of procedures are certainly where the money is. I could not care less and would even congratulate them if they were doing a lot of holistic healing, but in my experience, this is not the case a majority of the time. Yet a holistic approach can provide a good living for many people and get a lot of patients well. There is no doubt that the big cars and the big houses are not owned by those who run holistic pain centers. Those things belong to the spine surgeons and pain doctors, we all know that. Still, holistic medicine is slowly starting to spread across the country. There are many holistic pain centers in San Francisco and in Canada. I have a lecturer coming from Canada in March to bring us up to date with their experience.

Dr. Kabat-Zinn was able to start a huge international clinic outside of Boston, so we know it can be done. I hope to bring him to a city in the future and tell us about what he has accomplished. His work on holistic pain is internationally known.

The patient entering a holistic pain center should be given a long questionnaire to fill out regarding the history of her pain. I would also give her a yellow pad and a pencil and encourage her to write out this story—the longer the better. The provider's opening words should be, "What's going on in your life?" not, "Where is your pain?" There are many modalities that could be available in the pain clinic, but I suggest you offer about ten to twenty and just be good at those. The main ones were discussed previously in this book.

As a provider, I would recommend advertising in newspapers and TV, making some CDs and DVDs, and writing books to give to patients, as well as suggesting well-known pain books. Unfortunately it is difficult to find holistic pain books. I've written a book, *The Fraud of Chronic Pain*. and I would read the book *Meditation and Healing*, by Jon Kabat-Zinn. I also give lectures frequently on the subject and provide brochures for referring doctors, especially psychiatrists. Wellness centers should have a website that can be accessed easily and should pass out information, maybe even e-mail potential patients. I send people to doctor's offices with brochures, and I develop CDs, DVDs, and books to educate the patient, the public, and fellow doctors.

A nonnarcotic approach is not an easy road, but it's the correct approach most of the time. Nobody dies from a holistic approach applied correctly to chronic pain. I think a mindful meditation class needs to be the center of every holistic approach. That's critical. In my book *The Fraud of Chronic Pain*, I have an excellent chapter on mindfulness; it's a wonderful tool to teach stress reduction, pain reduction, etc.

Holistic, mindful medicine is the future. Practitioners of this kind of medicine will at first be ignored, then attacked, and finally others will say they knew it all along. I heard CEO John Mackey say that about his Whole Foods stores, and I think it applies equally to holistic medicine. Incidentally, I am one hundred percent convinced that John Mackey feels the same about what I'm doing. He sent me an e-mail saying that if you can shop at his stores, you will live a long time.

The Pain Industrial Complex: The Pain Barons

In 2002, OxyContin sales topped $1 billion for Purdue Pharma in spite of all the street activity having dried up because of government action. So where is the $1 billion in sales coming from? Doctor prescriptions and pain centers remain the biggest supplier. A significant number of those medications are sold on the street for $40 to $80 a pill, sometimes more. That's where the money is—people will do anything to get the prescription, and that is what the definition of addiction is: willingness to break the law to get the drug.

A lawyer from Chicago told me recently pain centers are charging $10,000 for injections in Chicago, and that's the key for unlocking the door to pick up a large narcotic prescription on a regular basis. It opens the door to the scripts and lifetime customers.

These are legal addicts. They don't have to buy the drug on the street now if they have the money and insurance. Unfortunately Medicaid pays for a lot of this. I know of a pain center in my area where ninety percent of the customers are on Medicaid. The government even pays for the taxi driver to take the recipient to the doctor and back. How sad! If this were stopped, we could save millions and maybe even a billion dollars a year in this country. Instead we are protecting the addict by giving him a narcotic under the protection of the law. We should give narcotics only for neuropathic pain or cancer pain. The majority of these patients are falsely diagnosed by the pain center. We need a new definition of pain.

It will be difficult to change the pain industry as there is too much money in it. Many of these doctors are making millions of dollars and the pharmaceutical companies are making billions a year, while addicts are on the street selling narcotics the government paid for. What a scam!

Summary

Pain: A New Definition

When you look at the whole problem of habituation and addiction, which turns normal people into opiate addicts and ruins lives, then you see the common enemy—the definition of what pain is! Is all the pain the same? A resounding no. Acute pain—a broken leg, heart attack, ruptured bowel, etc.—may require a short-term opioid. That's ten percent of the pain problems. These have an endpoint. Chronic pain, pain that lasts more than a month, is where the trouble is. Chronic pain is divided into neuropathic (twenty percent), nociceptive (ten percent), and what I call metabolic Pain (centralized brain pain) (seventy percent). All pain syndromes should be divided into these terms. We need to know what we are treating, that's critical! Pain is not a diagnosis, it's a symptom. The majority of providers are prescribing opiates and opioids for people with unclear, idiopathic, metabolic, central brain pain and that is a major mistake. It must stop! These providers are habituating and addicting a lot of people, resulting in many disabled adults and children and ruined lives. Certainly you can use opiates and opioids for cancer or clear-cut nerve damage pain, but not for things like tendonitis, bursitis, and degenerative disc disease. These can be treated with much more benign medication and holistic treatment methods like exercise, massage, and yoga. If the patient has non-malignant pain and the cause is unknown, the long-term use of prescription opiates or opioids should be avoided. Just because the patient says his level of pain is an eight, this should not mandate treatment. The health care provider needs to know the cause of the pain. Instead we are addicting a nation. We are a "pain nation." The industrial complex of pain societies, the quick fixers, the moneymakers, the pain centers, and overprescribing providers have addicted us and have taken us over. It's a war! Just recently I read another article explaining that pain centers moved to Georgia from Florida because Florida law became a lot stricter. OxyContin prescriptions are down ninety seven percent in Florida because of the strong state laws.

Nobody dies from pain, but many people die from pain medication. Pain doesn't kill; the treatment is killing us through complications leading to disability and death. Even children are being addicted. I doubt the medical society will lead the charge against this travesty, although I've tried in my town.

Medicaid is paying for most of this. Costs are heading into the billions and may double in five years or less. That's over a billion dollars going to patients and providers, paying for medicine, procedures, and free taxi rides to and from pain centers, resulting in disability, lost work, and ruined lives.

I propose a new definition of pain. Medicaid shouldn't pay for opioids or opiates for non-malignant metabolic Pain (centralized brain pain). If it didn't, a lot of these pain centers would close. This would save a lot of money and a lot of lives, and result in better treatment of pain problems. Some in the legislature are demanding that pain patients be referred to a pain center to help solve the problem, but this is like letting the fox into the chicken coop. It will not solve this problem, it will only make it worse. Medicaid should audit about two months' worth of books in a significant number of the pain centers, some of which I could name for them. The patients certainly know who they are; they have identified the overprescribing providers. Medicaid is the only organization that has the power to effect change; the other federal agencies need to go through a lot more red tape. But the legislature is slow to act because of the industrial complex. For example, the state of Georgia came one vote short of passing a new state law reforming opioid prescriptions, which would have saved a lot of lives.

All providers need to be paid better for the initial doctor visit so that talking pays, and the choice to go to the pain doctor might be reconsidered. Dumping the pain patients somewhere else does not solve the problem and often results in disability and death. We're all guilty—the patient who wants a quick fix, the patient who needs the dopamine and serotonin because of their horribly stressed-out lives, the doctor in the horrible money-making pain clinic who has no time and instead quickly injects the patient and prescribes unnecessary procedures and medications, all in the name of money. We need a new definition of pain, and to manage pain through things like stress reduction, exercise, diet, massage, yoga, tai chi, chiropractic visits, music therapy, and some "dancing with the stars." Insurance needs to help pay for this or it may never happen!

MORE RESOURCES FROM RUDY KACHMANN M.D.

Books:

Pain: We Need a New Definition
The Fraud of Chronic Pain
Healing Cancer with The Power Of Your Mind
Live to Be 100 with a Sound Mind and Body
The Call of Life
The Fraud of Alzheimer's Disease (also available on DVD)
Nocebo: Placebo's Evil Twin (also available on DVD and CD)
The Secret of the Non Diet for Adults (also available on DVD and CD)
The Secret of the Non Diet for Children (also available on DVD and CD)
Kid Scripts: Just What the Doctor Ordered
The Psychology of Eating (also available on DVD and CD)
Reversing Type 2 Diabetes in 60 Days (also available on DVD and CD)
Welcome to Your Mind Body (also available on DVD and CD)
Secrets of Motivating Yourself to Wellness (also available on DVD and CD)
For more titles, visit www.amazon.com.

DVDs:

The Mind and Stress (also available on CD)
Living Healthier and Longer (also available on CD)
Chinese Medicine (also available on CD)
Acute and Chronic Pain (also available on CD)
Smoking Cessation (also available on CD)
True Vitality (DVD only)
Secrets of the Mind and Cancer (DVD only)
For more titles, visit www.amazon.com.

Rudy Kachmann, M.D.

Renowned Medical Expert, Author, Lecturer, National and Internationally recognized Keynote speaker, Famed Neurosurgeon, TV Host, and Medical Director of the Kachmann Mind Body Institute.

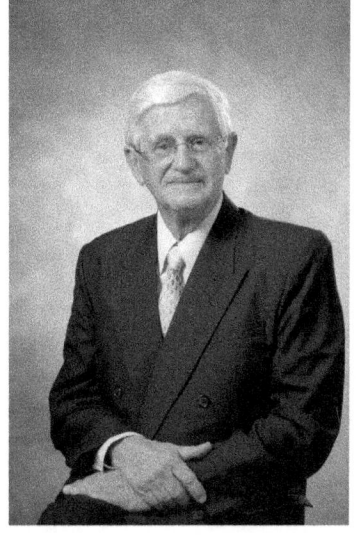

Dr. Rudy Kachmann's accomplishments are numerous. Dr. Kachmann has received numerous awards. Dr. Kachmann has authored books, Magazine publications, Medical books, DVDs and audio CDs. Dr. Kachmann

has appeared on network morning, noon, and evening news programs. In addition to these appearances Dr. Kachmann has filmed and appeared on PBS.

Dr. Kachmann is a passionate, wise and caring healer who is committed to helping people transforms their lives by showing them how to rise above their limitations, remove their roadblocks, rekindle their dreams, and transform their life by helping them understand their "whole person" connection. He is dedicated to making a difference in people's lives by explaining to them the importance of the Mind, Body and Spirit Connection.

Dr. Kachmann's years of experience as a neurosurgeon is critical to helping people learn the importance of how to avoid the huge cost of medical care, dangerous and unnecessary medications, injections, and surgeries.

Keynote Speaker Topics:

- Mind/Body/Spirit
- Health and Wellness
- Lifestyle
- Work/ Health and Life Balance

- Stress Management
- Exercise and Nutrition
- Healthy weight loss
- Corporate wellness motivator

Rudy Kachmann, M.D.

Kachmann Mind Body Institute
www.kachmannmindbody.com

www.ingramcontent.com/pod-product-compliance
Lightning Source LLC
Chambersburg PA
CBHW051509170526
45166CB00001B/460